D1331567

13
393

94

Caring for the Diabetic Patient

J. Kinson
SRN RCNT
Clinical Nurse Specialist in Diabetes, General Hospital, Birmingham

M. Nattrass
MB PhD MRCP
Consultant Physician, General Hospital, Birmingham and Senior
Clinical Lecturer, University of Birmingham

With contributions by

M.G. FitzGerald
MD FRCP
Consultant Physician, General Hospital, Birmingham and Senior
Clinical Lecturer, University of Birmingham

A.D. Wright
MB FRCP
Senior Lecturer in Medicine, University of Birmingham and
Honorary Consultant Physician, General Hospital, Birmingham

Foreword by
John M. Malins
Honorary Consultant Physician, The General Hospital,
Birmingham. Emeritus Professor of Medicine in the University of
Birmingham. Linacre Fellow, Royal College of Physicians of
London

Churchill Livingstone

EDINBURGH LONDON MELBOURNE AND NEW YORK 1984

CHURCHILL LIVINGSTONE
Medical Division of Longman Group Limited

Distributed in the United States of America by Churchill Livingstone Inc., 1560 Broadway,
New York, N. Y. 10036, and by associated companies, branches and representatives
throughout the world.

First published 1984

ISBN 0 443 02624 6

British Library Cataloguing in Publication Data
Kinson, J.M.
    Caring for the diabetic patient.
    1. Diabetes—Nursing
    I. Title   II. Nattrass, M.
    610.73'69   RC660

Library of Congress Cataloging in Publication Data
Kinson, J.
    Caring for the diabetic patient.
    Bibliography: p.
    Includes index.
    1. Diabetes—Nursing.   2. Nurse and patient.
    I. Nattrass, M.   II. Title.   [DNLM: 1. Diabetes mellitus—Nursing.
    WY 155 K56c]
    RC660.K53   1984   616.4'62   83-14424

Printed in Hong Kong by Sheck Wah Tong Printing Press Ltd.

Foreword

As a house physician in 1940 nothing made me more uneasy than the admission of a diabetic patient. I had been taught very little about diabetes and nothing about its management. Few of the nursing staff were more fortunate, but I was at least able to call for help from an experienced medical registrar. I had an uncomfortable feeling that some of these patients knew more about diabetes than I did and that they recognised my ignorance. Alas, the house physicians and nurses of today are not much better off. Diabetic Clinics are now recognised as necessary in every district hospital and their patients tend to remain under the care of the physician in charge, whether as in- or out-patient. In other parts of the hospital, diabetic patients are often quite a rarity and it is possible for medical students or student nurses to have no practical experience of diabetes at the bedside unless they are attached to the physician who runs the diabetic clinic.

Here is the book which fills that gap and does much more besides, a book which everyone from physician to junior student, from Senior Nursing Officer to most junior nurse can read with profit and enjoyment. The emphasis is on the need to train the patient in a sensible and practical attitude to his life-long fellow traveller. Always there is recognition of the fallibility of doctors, nurses and the diabetic patients for whom they care—and that has not been sufficiently understood in most of the writing on this subject. To combine a wholly up-to-date scientific approach with the broad traditional view (always up-to-date) of the care of diabetic patients is a rare feat.

One conclusion which has to be drawn is that the integration of the hospital service with those of the community and primary care is still a long way off. Attempts to organise a combined service for diabetic patients have only succeeded when a dedicated physician has kept alive the enthusiasm of hospital staff and general practitioners. But this must remain the objective.

J.M.M.

Preface

All nurses will encounter a diabetic patient at some time in their nursing career. The disease is common, presents in a variety of ways, and is life-long. It often seems that so much can go wrong with the diabetic patient that a feeling of anxiety is a normal response. Throughout medicine, such sensations invariably arise from ignorance.

It is our intention in writing this book to allay these fears by setting out simply the many aspects of diabetes. In order to do this we have attempted to deal with the disease and its problems as they arise in the patient and in the nurse/patient relationship. A second, equally important approach has been adopted. It is our belief that knowledge of the disease and the problems it poses is necessary for an understanding of the effects upon the patient and is essential to the caring role of the nurse.

The chapters of the book reflect this approach. A section on biochemistry highlights the differences between types of diabetes, and provides a basic understanding of how to deal with patients with an infection or teetering on the brink of ketoacidosis. The aetiology and natural history of the disease bring home the threat to health which it carries.

Diagnosis may well seem the province of the doctor but this would only be a partial truth. Thousands of diabetic patients owe their diagnosis, treatment, and good health to the nurse performing that most routine of all chores—urine testing. After diagnosis comes treatment. Much of the working lives of all of us is spent persuading and cajoling patients to follow treatment, and if we fail to understand the principles and importance of treatment this is all too readily conveyed to the patient, making our task doubly difficult.

Despite our efforts in diagnosis and treatment, the long-term complications of diabetes continue to be a major health problem. Knowledge of how complications arise and identification are important prerequisites for treatment and support of these patients.

The effective organisation of diabetic care both within and outside the hospital, and the role of the nurse in this, cannot be over-estimated in view of the sheer numbers of patients involved and the importance of careful follow-up.

In the introductory chapter we have emphasised the importance of education and the central role of the nurse. Later in the book this is amplified, indicating how patients learn and what they should be taught in order to enhance and prolong good health.

Finally, diabetic patients are, of course, individuals. Some develop the disease in childhood, some have pregnancies, and some have special problems in coming to terms with the disorder. In a similar manner, loosely defined groups of patients such as the elderly or ethnic minorities require us to modify our approach to the patient.

It is our experience from organising and participating in courses and study days for nurses involved in caring for diabetic patients that they need and demand knowledge and information to aid them in this work. We fervently hope that this book provides it and that ultimately it will help in Caring for the Diabetic Patient.

Birmingham   J.K.
1984   M.N.

Acknowledgements

Throughout this book we have quoted from the experience and studies of many of our colleagues. In addition to specific acknowledgement in the text we thank the following— Professor George Alberti, Dr Robert Tattersall, Dr Patrick Thorn, Dr Tom Hayes, Dr Ron Hill, Dr Peter Watkins, Dr Paul Rayner, and Ms Caroline Hitchen.

We would like to thank Mr Harry Buglass of the University of Birmingham and the Department of Clinical Illustration of the General Hospital, Birmingham, for the figures. The colour plates have been made possible through a generous grant from Novo Laboratories Limited for which we are grateful. The manuscript was typed by Mrs J. Merriman and Mrs R. Darling.

Finally, we would like to thank the Birmingham Hospital Saturday Fund who first gave financial impetus to the experience which this book reflects.

Contents

Introduction: the role of the nurse in caring for the diabetic patient

During this century, remarkable progress has been made in the knowledge and understanding of diabetes mellitus. The impetus arose from the discovery of insulin and its first use as a therapeutic agent in the 1920s. Few of the readers of this book will be able to recall the horrors of diabetes in the pre-insulin era and we must rely upon written descriptions of the disease. The second century Greek physician, Aretaeus paints a vivid picture of the nature of diabetes which was as true in 1900 as it was in his own time when he wrote '. . . a melting down of flesh and limbs into urine . . . life is disgusting and painful'. The debilitating illness was invariably followed, in those patients who today we would call insulin-dependent, by death in ketoacidosis.

With the isolation of insulin, mortality from this cause fell dramatically but it soon became clear that diabetes was not cured. The price of survival in many patients was the development of specific, disabling, long-term complications of diabetes. At present these remain major sources of chronic ill-health in diabetic patients and the avoidance is of major concern, not only to the patient, but to all who care for the diabetic patient.

In achieving this aim two factors create difficulty. Firstly, and as with many diseases, early detection is important before biochemical changes have resulted in permanent tissue damage. Secondly, despite advances in treatment it has proved extraordinarily difficult to control the biochemical abnormalities. Obtaining and maintaining, for long periods of time, normal blood glucose levels in diabetic patients has proved a most elusive goal.

Traditionally treatment has been the responsibility of the professional and we have been slow to realise the major role in the treatment of chronic disease that can be played by the patient. Gradually it has dawned on us that the diabetic patient is not simply a passive receiver of health-care but has an active part to play in his or her own management. For the patient to assume this role, however, correct education is of paramount importance, and it is as a direct consequence of this need that the role of the nurse in caring for the diabetic patient has developed enormously over the past decade. It is the nurse who has assumed more and more responsibility for patient education.

In this respect the creation of two posts has played a major part. The diabetes liaison nurse has forged a valuable link between the hospital-based physician and the community, allowing the patient to be seen as an individual within a family unit, while in recent years we have seen the emergence of nurse specialists in diabetes. This so-called extended role of the nurse has evolved gradually from its beginning in the United States of America in the mid 1950s.

Initially Britain lagged behind in this development. Nursing in the United Kingdom opted to develop along managerial lines and there appeared to be little scope for the nurse to develop her clinical skills. In 1971, the Royal College of Nursing set up a working party to discuss and define the role of the clinical nurse specialist. The outcome of their deliberations was a recommendation for the establishment of clinical nurse specialist posts for nurses considered expert practitioners, with considerable knowledge, a high degree of skill, and extensive experience in the speciality concerned.

One immediate danger was that the introduction of such a specialist nurse could be seen as a threat to the established order, but it was intended from the outset that the clinical nurse specialist should not detract from the authority and clinical expertise of the ward sister or the experienced community nurse or health visitor, but rather augment their skills and so increase the standard of care. The specialist nurse was to be, and today is, practitioner, teacher, co-ordinator, investigator, and innovator.

With a life-long disorder such as diabetes the scope for this role is tremendous. Specific tasks for the clinical nurse specialist in diabetes include: the follow-up of newly diagnosed patients with assessment of the family and identification of real and potential problems and the planning of future care; initiation, participation in, and continuation of patient and family education; and attendance at adult and/or paediatric clinics to discuss specific problems with the doctor and nursing colleagues, and to be present in an advisory capacity for patients and relatives. In addition, liaison with para-medical staff, particularly dieticians, chiropodists, social workers and psychologists; visits to places of work or educational establishments to discuss the needs of the diabetic patient with factory personnel, teachers and catering staff; and ready accessibility for patients or parents of diabetic children in times of emergency and stress are all areas of involvement of the clinical nurse specialist.

It must be considered unlikely that large numbers of these posts will be established in view of competition for resources, and we must consider carefully how best to use the time and talents of the clinical nurse specialist in diabetes. Individual patient and family education will clearly be an important part of the job but concentration upon a small number of patients is always at the expense of the majority. An extended role for the clinical nurse specialist, therefore, must include the education of colleagues with the setting up of study days for hospital and community nurses, and lecturing to student nurses, community nurses and health visitors in training.

Many diabetic units throughout the United Kingdom are setting up study days for nurses, often generously aided by industrial sponsorship. It is likely that the nurse whose day to day job involves the care of the diabetic patient will be called upon to play a greater part in the education of her colleagues, yet little attention is paid to preparing her for this role. Many eminent lecturers would admit that they had received no formal instruction on how to teach or, more specifically, how people learn. It is presumed that the physician and the nurse specialising in diabetes can teach, but regrettably this is not always the case. Perhaps it should be mandatory for the nurse involved in patient and colleague education to take the City and Guilds of London Institute Course—'The Further Education Teachers' Certificate'. This part-time course provides an introduction to the psychology of learning and lesson planning, and provides the opportunity for observed teaching practice.

Fortunately, more and more opportunities are opening up for further education. The British Diabetic Association has a professional services section which caters for nursing and paramedical staff, and more recently the Joint Board of Clinical Nursing Studies has established a short course in diabetes for trained nurses.

We should acknowledge, however, that concentration upon a 'specialist' may evoke a firm reaction in the many other staff who care for their diabetic patients. The nurse specialist is still a comparatively rare breed and most patients with diabetes receive their care and education by hospital ward staff or by community nurses.

Nursing in diabetes emphasises the caring role of the nurse and Peplau's definition of nursing epitomises the role of the nurse in diabetes 'a unique human relationship between an individual who is sick or in need of health services and a nurse specially educated to recognise and respond to the need for help. Nursing is an education instrument, a maturing force, that aims in the direction of creative, constructive, personal and community living'. What follows in this book is intended for all nurses who care for the diabetic patient, for hospital staff and community nurses as much as for the clinical nurse specialist, in the hope that it will help the nurse achieve these goals.

1

The biochemistry, aetiology and natural history of diabetes

BLOOD GLUCOSE

Introduction

In a normal person blood glucose concentration does not vary very much over the course of 24 hours. There are good biological reasons why this should be so. It must be remembered that our ancestors were hunters and had to make the most of their abilities and their sometimes sporadic meals. A rise in the blood glucose concentration to the level at which glucose appears in the urine would result in loss of valuable and often hard earned calories. Man who could avoid this would therefore be in an advantageous position. At the other extreme, since normal brain function depends upon a supply of glucose via the blood, a lowering of this supply by a fall in blood glucose leads to poor cerebral function—the features of hypoglycaemia. The effects of such episodes upon man the hunter, would be devastating not only in a deterioration of his skills as a hunter but possibly in turning him from predator into prey. The ability to keep blood glucose concentration within narrow limits, therefore, has evolved through being advantageous to the human organism.

Regulation of blood glucose concentration?

How is blood glucose concentration kept within these narrow limits? It is a general rule applicable to all substances in the blood that the final concentration of the substance is the balance between the amount produced by the body plus the amount derived from outside sources, and the amount removed from blood and used. Thus at a given point in time, a person's blood glucose concentration represents the balance between the amount obtained from meals and the amount produced, versus the amount extracted from the blood by cells for utilisation.

Dietary supply

Firstly, we shall consider glucose which is obtained from meals.

This is perhaps the easiest of the three parts of the process to understand. Carbohydrates in food are broken down (digested) in the stomach. Many of the carbohydrates in food are termed 'complex carbohydrates' such as starch from potatoes or rice. In complex carbohydrates the sugars are bonded together. There is a major advantage to the consumer when eating complex carbohydrate since absorption of complex carbohydrate takes longer and spreading absorption over a longer period of time helps to maintain the constancy of the blood glucose concentration. It can be easily shown that if the same amount of apples, for example, are eaten as apple juice, stewed apple, or the original fruit, the patterns of absorption are very different with juice absorbed rapidly and the whole fruit slowest of the three. The same amount is absorbed but the time over which it is absorbed varies considerably. This spreading of absorption with time is advantageous in making less demands upon the mechanisms which help to regulate the blood glucose concentration. Having broken down the complex carbohydrates in the gut they can be absorbed. Where do they go and for what are they used?

Few people in the western world do not know where the next meal is coming from or, perhaps more importantly, when it will be. Returning to the consideration of our ancestor, man the hunter, his lifestyle was very different and his next meal depended upon a successful effort for prey. This might mean for him a period of days without food during which time his brain needed a steady supply of glucose supplied by the blood, and at the kill he might have to call upon reserves of energy for muscles in a strenuous fight.

One of the major tasks of nutrient supply by meals is to lay down these reserves in order to maintain blood glucose during fasting, and supply energy quickly and in large amounts when needed. Thus a considerable proportion of each meal is laid down in reserve. A major storage compound is glycogen. Most cells contain some glycogen but only in liver and muscle is it able to fulfil the roles mentioned above. Glycogen is a polymer of glucose. This simply means that it consists of many glucose

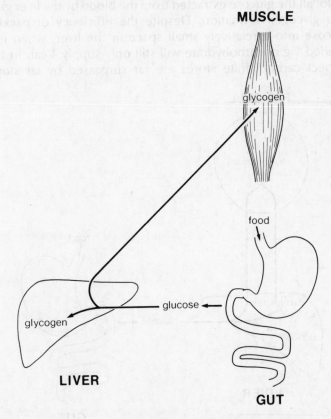

Figure 1.1 Storage in liver and muscle of glucose obtained from meals.

residues joined together chemically. Now, given a set of 'lego'
a child may join together thirty pieces in a single line to stretch
from the corner of the lounge to the kitchen (and may simultaneously incur the wrath of the rest of the family). Alternatively, the child can use up a small corner of the lounge by
joining thirty pieces of lego six pieces long by five pieces high.
This more sensible use of space is how glucose is stored as
glycogen. Absorption of sugars from the gut is by the portal
blood system and the liver is ideally placed in this system to
extract and store glucose. About 60 per cent of glucose
absorbed is handled in this way. The remainder passes through
the liver and is available to other tissues for storage and for
utilisation (Fig. 1.1).

Not all the glucose extracted from the blood by the liver goes
into glycogen formation. Despite the efficiency of packing
glucose into a relatively small space in the liver, when it is
needed 1 g of carbohydrate will still only supply 4 cal. In this
respect carbohydrate stores are far surpassed by fat stores

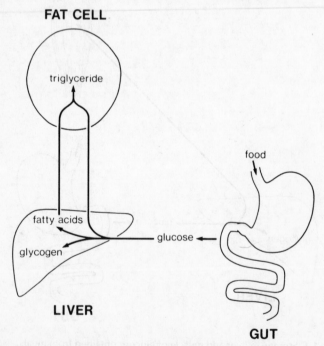

Figure 1.2 Storage in liver and fat cells of glucose obtained from meals.

which yield 9 cal per gram. Some of our fat stores come from dietary supply of fat but the remainder is synthesised mainly by the liver. The liver can start with glucose and by fairly elaborate metabolic pathways produce cholesterol, fatty acids, and triglycerides. Thus, starting with glucose entering the liver after meals some of it will find its way into storage fat in the fat cell. It is helped in this respect by the glucose which escapes the liver and arrives at the fat cell, some of this being incorporated into triglyceride—the storage fat (Fig. 1.2).

To fully round off the benefits of meals the dietary supply of protein should be considered. Proteins are digested to their constituent building blocks, amino acids. After absorption these can be re-built into body proteins and there is a constant demand upon the body to synthesise new proteins for old. Many functional varieties of proteins exist, some maintain our structure, some are highly specialised such as enzymes and hormones and some have relatively little function such as hair and toe nails. All have one thing in common and that is that they 'turnover' albeit at varying rates. Greater structural demands of course, as in the growth spurt of adolescence or during pregnancy, lead to greater demands upon dietary supply of amino acids. Storage proteins also have a role to play, as we will see later in this section in helping prop-up the blood glucose concentration during fasting.

Summary. Dietary supply of complex nutrients, fats, proteins, and carbohydrates leads after digestion and absorption to synthesis of substances for long-term use e.g. structural proteins, and to deposition of storage compounds such as glycogen and triglyceride for use by the organism in the fasting state.

Maintaining blood glucose during fasting

Having considered supply of nutrients by meals, particularly glucose supply, and its deposition in storage forms we can now consider what happens during fasting.

An important concept to grapple with is that of fasting. Earlier it was mentioned that how you eat apples is important in the time over which they are absorbed. Whichever form they are eaten in, however, absorption is finished by two hours and this applies to most of the meals we eat. Of course at a

Henry VIII style banquet we may actually eat for longer than two hours but few hospital staff canteens go in for sucking pig or wild boar and the rapid, not to say frantic way, in which hospital staff eat—a readily observable fact—allows us to predict with some certainty that within two hours absorption will be complete. After two hours therefore, the organism must change from trying to keep blood glucose down following meals, to attempting to keep it up. This is the hall-mark of the fasting state and since few people eat at two hourly intervals we are in the fasting state for a considerable part of the day and certainly for most of the night. Thus, the fasting state which is referred to is *not* the prolonged fast of a hunger striker but a substantial part of the 24 hours of most people. With this in mind the following discussion will be confined to what happens after an overnight fast with the proviso that at other times during a 24-hour cycle the same rules are applicable.

After an overnight fast two processes contribute to main-taining blood glucose concentration. The first, which is prob-ably responsible for approximately 75 per cent, is the breakdown of glycogen stored in the liver (Fig. 1.3). The liver contains all the enzymes involved in conversion of glycogen to glucose and the latter is released into the blood. It should be noted that this does not occur from glycogen stored in muscle. Muscle glycogen is available for energy production through breakdown in situ but lacks a vital enzyme for glucose production and release. A normal liver can store about 120 g of glycogen and since 1 g will yield 4 cal the total calorific value of these stores is only about 500 cal. Thus, while in short-term fasting glycogen is important, stores are rapidly diminished if

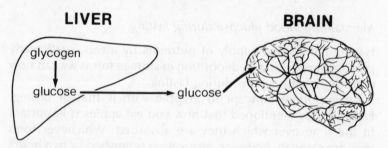

LIVER   **BRAIN**

glycogen
↓
glucose ⟶ glucose

Figure 1.3 The source of glucose used by brain during fasting.

fasting is prolonged. During prolonged fasting, and to supply the remaining 25 per cent of blood glucose after an overnight fast, a second pathway is used. In this second pathway glucose is synthesised by the liver, and to a much lesser extent by the kidney. The process is known as gluconeogenesis. (It should be noted that many of the terms used in metabolism become clearer if broken into their constituent parts e.g. gluco, neo, genesis.)

The process of gluconeogenesis is extremely difficult to define. Traditional teaching has it that gluconeogenesis is synthesis of glucose from non-carbohydrate sources, particularly from protein. Unfortunately, advances in biochemistry have suggested that this is not totally true. If the term must be defined then a simple definition would be as follows. The compound glucose is made up of carbon, hydrogen and oxygen. There are six carbons in each glucose molecule. Gluconeogenesis is the synthesis of glucose, the six carbon compound from smaller substances containing three or four carbons.

An alternative way to think of gluconeogenesis is that it is a form of recycling of carbon. The starting blocks for synthesis are four major compounds—lactate, pyruvate, alanine and glycerol (Fig. 1.4). Although glucose synthesis occurs in the liver these compounds come from other tissues and get to the liver in the blood. If we consider pyruvate and lactate firstly, these two compounds are produced when glucose is broken

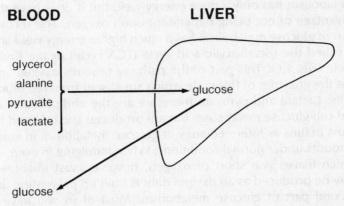

Figure 1.4 Gluconeogenesis.

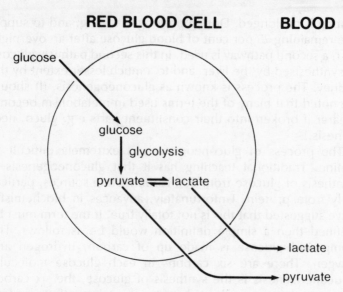

RED BLOOD CELL   **BLOOD**

glucose

glucose

glycolysis

pyruvate $\rightleftharpoons$ lactate

lactate

pyruvate

Figure 1.5 Glucose breakdown in red blood cells.

down by a tissue such as muscle, red blood cells, kidney, nervous tissue etc. In some of these tissues, particularly red blood cells, glucose metabolism ends at pyruvate and lactate since they lack the essential enzymes for further metabolism (Fig. 1.5). This first part of glucose metabolism, the breakdown of glycogen or glucose to pyruvate or lactate is called glycolysis, or after the people who originally described the pathway, the Embden-Myerhoff-Parnas pathway. This part of glucose metabolism has only a poor energy yield but it does have the advantage of not being dependent upon oxygen. The second part of glucose metabolism has a much higher energy yield and is called the tricarboxylic acid cycle (TCA cycle) or the Krebs cycle (Fig. 1.6). This part of the pathway requires oxygen and it is the enzymes of this cycle which are absent from red blood cells. Lactate and pyruvate therefore are the end-products of red cell glucose metabolism but are produced and released by most tissues as intermediaries of glucose metabolism in small amounts under normal conditions. When indulging in exercise which leaves you short of oxygen, however, vast quantities may be produced as an oxygen debt is built up preventing the second part of glucose metabolism. Most of us will have a marked rise in blood lactate concentration due to production

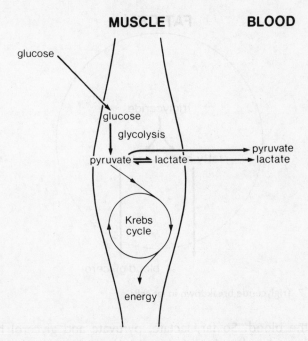

Figure 1.6 Glucose breakdown in muscle.

and release from muscles during a strenuous game of squash. At the extreme, during top-class 100 metre sprinting when the athlete draws probably one to two breaths only, large quantities of lactate are released into the blood. For most of us walking or jogging or running to a cardiac arrest would raise blood lactate, but the important point is that small amounts of pyruvate and lactate are released from tissues continuously, the amounts rising with other features of a normal life.

If the accent in the above discussion appears to be on lactate, that is only because quantitatively it is more important than pyruvate with the lactate concentration in blood being about ten times that of pyruvate during normal conditions.

In a similar manner glycerol is not quantitatively as important as lactate. Glycerol is produced by the breakdown of triglycerides (Fig. 1.7). Indeed triglyceride is only a combination of fatty acids (3—hence the prefix tri-) and glycerol. When energy is required from stores of triglyceride, fatty acids and glycerol are released and both are transported to the liver. The liver is the only organ in man that can extract and use glycerol

FAT CELL

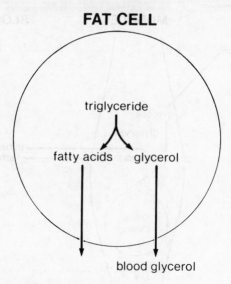

Figure 1.7 Triglyceride breakdown in fat cells.

from the blood. So far, lactate, pyruvate and glycerol have been considered—what of alanine? Alanine is an amino acid and contributes significantly to glucose production in the liver. Small amounts of other amino acids also contribute but it can be shown that alanine released by muscles exceeds the release of other amino acids. It is probable that this is the source of the definition of gluconeogenesis as synthesis of glucose from amino acids which, as was stated earlier, is not an entirely adequate definition. The reason for this is as follows:

If muscle is broken down chemically and the amount of each amino acid analysed it can be calculated that under normal conditions the release of alanine from muscle is out of all proportion to the muscle content. Implicit in this finding is the idea that alanine must be synthesised in muscle before being released into the blood and recent evidence supports this. Indeed, pyruvate and alanine have similar chemical structures with the latter having an amino group (i.e. a nitrogen-containing group). It now appears that breakdown of muscle protein releasing other amino acids is followed by donation of their nitrogen groups to pyruvate with resultant alanine formation (Fig. 1.8). The carbon skeleton of amino acids which is left is utilised and alanine really functions as a transport

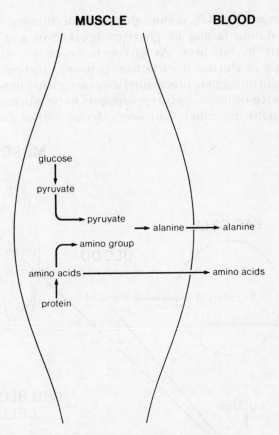

Figure 1.8 Partial breakdown of glucose and protein in muscle.

substance from muscle to liver for nitrogen. When these compounds are taken into the liver the nitrogen is split from alanine reforming pyruvate. The 3-carbon compounds are than used in glucose synthesis and this complex enzymic process is the one termed 'gluconeogenesis'.

Thus it can be seen that formation of glucose from lactate, pyruvate, glycerol and alanine is really a recycling since the carbon framework was originally derived from glucose. The glucose-lactate-glucose cycle is called the Cori cycle after the husband and wife team who were the first to describe this cycle. Apart from the recycling of carbon, net production of glucose, that is production of new glucose, only occurs from the small amounts of other amino acids released from muscle.

Summary (Fig. 1.9). Blood glucose concentration is maintained during fasting by glycogen breakdown and glucose synthesis in the liver. As glycogen stores are exhausted synthesis of glucose from lactate, pyruvate, alanine and glycerol (gluconeogenic precursors) assumes greater importance. The source of these precursors appears to be glucose metabolism in tissues other than liver. Under normal conditions

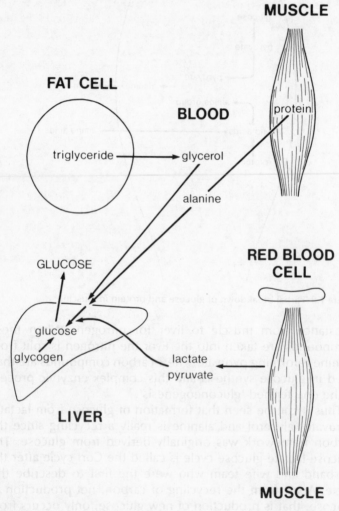

Figure 1.9 Summary: maintenance of the blood glucose concentration.

other amino acids contribute little to glucose formation but are of greater importance in some states, e.g. during prolonged fasting or during acidosis. Glycerol from triglycerides is used in gluconeogenesis. Fatty acids although originally derived from glucose in part, cannot be made into glucose.

Uptake and use of glucose by tissues

We have already to a large extent covered the extraction of glucose from the blood and its utilisation. The liver extracts glucose and uses it to synthesise glycogen and fatty acids. Most tissues, however, require glucose to a greater or a lesser extent. As glucose in the blood passes round the body it is taken out of the blood by other tissues and used mainly to produce energy to maintain vital activities of the cells of those tissues. The first step in this process is glucose uptake by the cells. Here there are two important differences between tissues. Certain tissues of which brain is a good example have a constant demand for glucose to maintain them in a viable state. The removal of glucose from the blood into the cells is not dependent upon the hormone insulin. In other tissues, however, such as muscle and fat, uptake of glucose from the blood into the cells is a process which depends upon adequate amounts of circulating insulin. This difference ensures that vital tissues such as brain are able to extract glucose from the blood in preference to other less demanding tissues.

Hormonal control of blood glucose concentration

For this system to function at maximum efficiency it must be carefully regulated. Clearly it would be a waste of resources if glucose production by the liver were to occur after meals when dietary supply of glucose is adequate. During feeding or during fasting the signal must go out delineating which state the organism is in. There is good evidence that both states are regulated and signalled by the hormone insulin—the fed state by a rise in insulin concentration, and the fasting state by a fall in circulating insulin.

Let us take as a starting point a person sitting down to eat a meal. It is known that anticipation of a meal increases secretion of insulin from the pancreas but the major surge follows the arrival of absorbed nutrients at the B cell. Circulating insulin concentrations rise and the increased concentration reaching the liver inhibits glucose production by shutting off both glycogen breakdown and gluconeogenesis. As concentrations of insulin continue to rise in the peripheral blood the hormone increases the entry of glucose into cells, particularly muscle and fat cells. In turn this leads to glucose metabolism. Not only is glycogen breakdown in liver stopped by insulin but storage of glycogen is stimulated. In contrast to muscle and fat cells where insulin is needed for entry of glucose, the liver cell, like cells of the brain, has no barrier to glucose entry and this simply occurs with the rise in glucose after a meal. As well as forming glycogen some of this glucose is directed to fat synthesis. Thus, the rise in insulin serves to prevent an excessive rise of glucose in the blood both by preventing production by the body and enhancing storage and utilisation.

The fall in circulating insulin also signals the change from the fed to the fasted state. As insulin concentrations decrease so glucose uptake by muscle and fat cells decreases. As insulin and blood glucose concentration decrease further, the inhibition on liver glucose production is relieved and from taking glucose out of the circulation after feeding, the liver changes to producing glucose to sustain the circulating concentration.

Thus both glucose production and glucose utilisation are regulated by insulin and since these determine blood glucose concentration the role of insulin in regulating this can be seen.

Other actions of insulin

Insulin has actions way beyond those upon carbohydrate metabolism. It is the major anabolic hormone in adults—that is it is the storage hormone par excellence. Insulin both stimulates protein synthesis and prevents protein breakdown. Again this cycle makes biological sense in that to maximise resources protein should be laid down in times of plenty (after feeding), and utilised when the going is rough. In addition insulin affects fat metabolism, and part of this has been touched on as it arose in the consideration of glucose metabolism. One other area of fat metabolism needs further consideration because of its importance in diabetes.

Neither the storage of fat nor its breakdown are simple

passive processes. It has already been stated that the liver synthesises fatty acids. Following synthesis three fatty acid units have a glycerol derivative bound to them and in this form (triglyceride) the liver releases them. After transport in the blood the triglyceride is presented to the fat cell. Before entry it is broken down and it is the fatty acids which enter the cell. Again triglyceride is formed by attachment of a glycerol derivative originating in glucose. Insulin affects what happens at the surface of the fat cell and also the uptake of glucose to make the glyceride part. High concentrations stimulate both processes so that after feeding fat is stored.

These reserves of fat can be called upon during fasting (Fig. 1.10). Triglyceride is broken down to glycerol which passes to the liver for glucose synthesis and fatty acids, which

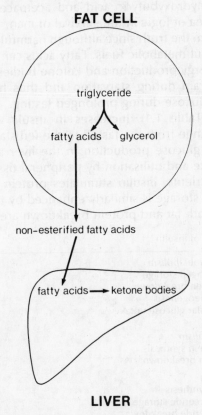

Figure 1.10 Source and production of ketone bodies.

when not bound to glycerol are termed non-esterified, are also taken up by the liver. Here they are broken down to supply energy and the final breakdown products are the ketone bodies, 3-hydroxybutyrate, acetoacetate and acetone. Liver uptake of fatty acids and hence ketone body formation is directly proportional to circulating concentration and thus the amount of ketone bodies formed is dependent upon the amount of fatty acids released by the fat cell. This breakdown of fat is termed lipolysis and the process is exquisitely sensitive to insulin. Increased concentrations of insulin after meals prevent fat breakdown while falling concentrations and low levels of insulin during fasting allow lipolysis.

On the face of it the production of fatty acids and ketone bodies which are apparently harmful compounds particularly the acids, 3-hydroxybutyric acid and acetoacetic acid, goes against the idea of logic in the survival of man. Nothing could be farther from the truth since although harmful in excess they are most useful metabolic fuels. Fatty acids can be utilised by muscle in energy production and ketone bodies can be metabolised by brain during starvation and thus have a sparing effect upon glucose during prolonged fasting.

Summary (Table 1.1). Increases in insulin concentration signal the change from the fasted to the fed state. The rise in insulin stops glucose production in the liver and stimulates glucose uptake and utilisation by peripheral tissues. With the supply of nutrients, insulin stimulates protein synthesis. Fat synthesis and storage is similarly enhanced by the increase in insulin and both fat and protein breakdown are stopped.

Table 1.1 Actions of insulin

a. *Carbohydrate metabolism*	
promotes glycogen storage	liver
inhibits glycogen breakdown	liver
inhibits gluconeogenesis	liver
promotes cellular glucose uptake	muscle
	fat cells
b. *Protein metabolism*	
promotes protein synthesis	muscle
inhibits protein breakdown	muscle
c. *Fat metabolism*	
promotes fat synthesis	liver
promotes triglyceride storage	fat cells
inhibits triglyceride breakdown	fat cells

The fall in insulin after nutrients have been utilised signals the change back to the fasting state. The low insulin concentrations have a permissive effect, allowing glucose production, fat breakdown and protein breakdown. At the same time the lack of insulin results in low levels of tissue uptake of glucose and poor fat and protein synthesis.

Catabolic hormones

While insulin is the major anabolic hormone during normal life its actions are opposed by a number of hormones collectively termed 'catabolic hormones'. These include glucagon, corticosteroids, and the catecholamines, adrenaline and noradrenaline. A detailed consideration of their metabolic effects is unnecessary but all act to break down stores and hence raise blood glucose concentration. This may occur through a direct effect, e.g. glucagon stimulates glycogen breakdown in the liver, or may occur through alterations in insulin secretion.

Just how important these hormones are in maintaining blood glucose concentration in normal life is difficult to say. What is apparent, however, is that during infection, trauma or other stress, concentrations of these hormones rise dramatically, enhancing the breakdown of glycogen and fat and thus the production of glucose and ketone bodies. We will return to this point later when considering the effects of surgery and/or infection in the diabetic patient and also the development of diabetic ketoacidosis.

Diabetes mellitus

Diabetes is characterised by deficiencies of insulin action. Whether this is due to an absolute deficiency of insulin with virtually no circulating insulin or to a short-fall in insulin requirement (relative deficiency) depends upon the type of diabetes (Ch. 2). At the cell level, however, the end result is similar. The clearest example is the newly diagnosed insulin-dependent diabetic and for an examination of the metabolic consequences we shall consider this case. Those readers who prefer active recall of facts to further passive reading would be well advised to pause at this stage and with pen and paper draw up a list of the effects of insulin upon metabolic pathways.

From there it is but a short step to deriving the effects of insulin deficiency.

Newly diagnosed insulin-dependent diabetic patients have very low levels of circulating insulin. The first question to answer is why blood glucose concentration is high. We started this section with a general statement that the concentration in the blood is a balance between production and utilisation. Insulin inhibits glucose production and promotes utilisation. In insulin deficiency, therefore, production of glucose is unchecked contributing to a rise in blood glucose, and utilisation is impaired. As feeding continues the absorbed glucose cannot be removed from the blood to any great extent and this further exacerbates the rise in blood glucose.

Secondly, we should ask what happens to protein metabolism. Here again the effect of insulin in stimulating protein synthesis and reducing breakdown is lost. In insulin deficiency there is poor synthesis of proteins and breakdown is relatively unchecked, all contributing to the wasted appearance of the newly diagnosed patient.

Thirdly, about 12 per cent of patients with diabetic ketoacidosis are newly diagnosed cases. The lack of insulin results in poor fat storage and enhanced breakdown contributing to the weight loss of the patient. The release of fatty acids is unchecked and hence ketone bodies are formed from breakdown in the liver. Since the ketone bodies are acids the full blown picture of diabetic ketoacidosis may follow.

This is the complete picture but lesser degrees will occur in all newly diagnosed diabetics. Yet the problem does not end there. We have seen how the insulin response to meals and the fall with fasting are sensitively linked to food intake or its lack. Our present insulin regimens for treating insulin-dependent diabetics are, by contrast, crude, depositing often large amounts of insulin in subcutaneous depots with fixed absorption patterns. The results upon metabolism are equivalent to coarse tuning on a television set. The fine tuning is lost and without the exquisite sensitivity it becomes difficult to maintain good metabolic control. We shall return to this point in Chapter 2.

In other types of diabetes similar principles apply. Understanding of the biochemical changes in non-insulin-dependent diabetics is hampered by uncertainty as to the cause of diabetes in such people. Whether due to insulin deficiency or insulin resistance is considered in the discussion on aetiology but the biochemical results of these two possibilities are similar—a relatively deficient action of insulin upon cells leading to hyperglycaemia.

Non-insulin-dependent diabetics, however, are 'ketosis-resistant'—that is they do not readily form ketone bodies. An important concept is that not all the metabolic effects of insulin require the same elevation of insulin concentration. Thus, fat breakdown is extremely sensitive to inhibition by insulin while cellular glucose uptake needs a high circulating concentration of insulin. Thus it may be argued in non-insulin-dependent diabetics that sufficient insulin (or insulin action) is present to inhibit ketone body formation but insufficient to stimulate removal of glucose from the blood.

Summary (Table 1.2). Lack of the effects of insulin in diabetes allows blood glucose concentration to rise by impairing utilisation and permitting liver production of glucose. In addition, the deficit affects protein metabolism allowing breakdown and impairing synthesis, and also fat metabolism allowing breakdown with consequent ketone body formation and impairing synthesis. The features are seen at their worst in newly diagnosed patients who need insulin, but occur in most diabetic patients on insulin at some time in the day or night when current therapies fail to achieve appropriate insulin concentrations.

Patients who are not insulin-dependent retain sufficient action of insulin to prevent excessive fat breakdown and hence do not develop ketoacidosis. There is insufficient insulin

Table 1.2 Consequences of insulin deficiency

1. *Carbohydrate metabolism*
   glycogen breakdown enhanced
   gluconeogenesis enhanced
   impaired glycogen storage
   impaired cellular uptake of glucose } ——→ hyperglycaemia

2. *Protein metabolism*
   protein breakdown
   impaired protein synthesis } ——→ wasting

3. *Fat metabolism*
   triglyceride breakdown
   impaired fat storage } ——→ ketosis
                          ——→ weight loss

activity at a cellular level to prevent a rise in blood glucose concentration.

Conclusion

The foregoing discussion has dealt with the metabolic effects of insulin. In all types of diabetes there is a deficient effect of insulin acting upon cells. The extent of the deficient effects of insulin, however, vary with different types of diabetes. The single unifying biochemical abnormality in diabetes is a raised blood glucose concentration. This allows diagnosis and is a means for monitoring the efficiencies of our various therapies. At certain times during our treatment of diabetes, for example in diabetic ketoacidosis or during the growth spurt of adolescence in a diabetic teenager, other aspects of the deficient action of insulin may assume greater importance.

AETIOLOGY AND TYPES OF DIABETES

Introduction

Diabetes mellitus is a heterogeneous disorder. As in anaemia where there may be a number of causes for the low haemoglobin, there may be a number of causes for the raised blood glucose in diabetes. Whether there is a single cause or a number of causes is unknown and while this remains so, trying to sort out subgroups of diabetes will have to depend upon other factors. For many years the two major subgroups were known as juvenile-onset and maturity-onset—that is, the division was largely based on the age at presentation. This subdivision also conveniently fitted the patterns of treatment, juvenile-onset with insulin treatment and maturity-onset with diet or oral agent treatment. It was readily apparent, however, that some young people with diabetes were not insulin-dependent, and rather more of mature years were insulin-dependent. Thus the subdivision did not hold for everyone. Recently new light on the aetiology of diabetes has led to a revision of the classification (Table 1.3). Type 1 diabetes replaced the older terms juvenile-onset or insulin-dependent,

Table 1.3 The heterogeneous nature of diabetes

Aetiological Type	Type 1	Type 2
Clinical onset	rapid	insidious
Genetic susceptibility	HLA-linked	present but unknown
Environmental factors	viruses	obesity stress drugs
Immunity	Islet cell antibodies	absent

and Type 2 replaced maturity-onset or non-insulin dependent, and, as will be seen, these terms are useful in a consideration of the aetiology in different subgroups. With a revision of the diagnostic criteria and classification by the World Health Organization came another classification. We can now return to insulin-dependent diabetes mellitus (IDDM); those patients not dependent upon insulin have non-insulin-dependent diabetes mellitus (NIDDM). If the reader is confused already he or she may take solace from the fact that they are not alone. Hopefully, clearer ideas will emerge as we chart the way through the minefield.

Insulin-dependent diabetes mellitus (IDDM)

A newly diagnosed child with diabetes mellitus does not usually arouse doubts as to which group of patients he or she fits into. This is especially so when the presentation is in diabetic ketoacidosis. From the biochemistry (p. 20) it can be deduced that the production of excessive amounts of ketone bodies is a clear marker of gross insulin deficiency. Other markers of this deficiency would include the burning of fat reserves to produce ketones and the breakdown of proteins. The two combine to make weight loss and wasting a prominent feature of the illness. What of the more traditional symptoms of thirst and polyuria? These reflect the prevailing blood glucose concentration. Once the latter rises above the renal threshold for glucose (about 10 mmol/l in most people) polyuria is inevitable since glucose is a diuretic. The human body does not function by excreting treacle, and water loss is obligatory with the glucose. It is the polyuria which leads to thirst and not, as many patients assume, that because they are drinking more they excrete more. These symptoms are, to a certain extent, dependent from this point on upon what is drunk to relieve the thirst, and the height of the blood glucose concentration may simply reflect quenching the thirst by glucose containing drinks. Thus, the height of the blood glucose concentration does not indicate one type of diabetes or another.

The need for insulin is usually assessed therefore on clinical grounds and except in ketoacidosis is usually a composite picture. From the clinical presentation it is inferred that insulin secretion is reduced due to damage to insulin-producing cells which is the basic pathological lesion in this type of diabetes.

Aetiology

What is known of possible causes of insulin-dependent diabetes mellitus?

In general terms the tendency for a person to develop a disease depends upon two factors—their genetic make-up or what they inherit, and what factors in the environment they come into contact with. Each disease fits into a spectrum from, for example, haemophilia which is entirely genetic to the common cold which is entirely of environmental origin. In determining the aetiology of insulin-dependent diabetes mellitus we should examine these two factors.

Genetic factors. Firstly, let us consider the genetics of this type of diabetes. In this respect the HLA system has thrown considerable light upon aetiology and the first consideration must be what this system is.

It is readily apparent that if you wish to transplant one organ from a human being to another human this cannot be done at random. In the majority of cases the transplanted organ would be recognised as foreign (i.e. not of self), attacked by the host's immune response and rejected. For more successful transplantation some degree of matching of donor and recipient must take place. This is so common for blood transfusion that we do not think twice about it, but failure to match blood groups before transfusion could have dire consequences. For organ transplantation it is insufficient simply to match up the blood groups of the two people involved. The organ may still be rejected.

Rejection of a transplanted organ occurs because there are antigens on the surface of cells in the transplanted organ and these antigens are determined by what is inherited. The 'major histo-compatibility system' in man is located on chromosome 6 and within this system lie the determinants of the major histo-compatibility antigens—the HLA system.

Each individual receives one chromosome 6 from each parent. On these two chromosomes are the loci which determine the specific antigens which will be present on cell surfaces. The HLA system is described as polymorphic which means that from each locus a number of antigens may result— for example the DR locus may determine the antigens DR1, DR2, DR3 etc to DR10. An individual, however, will only have one of these for each chromosome, e.g. DR3 from one chromosome and DR4 from the other.

For reasons which are not clear, certain antigens occur more commonly in the general population than others but provided we take a large enough population the frequency of an antigen in normal subjects can be calculated. The next step is to look at the genetic make-up of insulin-dependent diabetic patients to see if the antigens occur with the same frequency. If the HLA antigens occur with the same frequency in insulin-dependent diabetic patients as in the normal population then we could conclude that the genetics of the HLA system had little or nothing to do with the development of the disease. If an antigen does not, we can calculate the risk of developing insulin-dependent diabetes if specific antigens are possessed.

There have been many studies of the HLA system in insulin-dependent diabetic patients. The picture that emerges is that some antigens do indeed occur more commonly in diabetic patients (Fig. 1.11). In other words an increased risk of developing diabetes is observed in subjects who possess the antigens HLA A1, A2, B8, B18, B15, B40, Dw3, Dw4, DR3, DR4. Current evidence suggests that the major determinants of the risk of diabetes are the antigens DR3 and DR4 and the finding that antigens of the A, B, Cw and Dw series seem implicated is because these particular antigens occur more commonly in association with DR3 and DR4.

We can go a little further than this statement by asserting

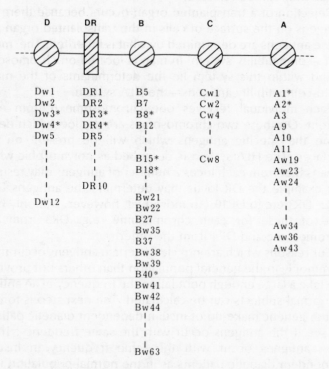

Figure 1.11 Chromosome 6: the relationship of the 5 series is shown. Each individual has one antigen determinant from each series per chromosome. The possible antigens are shown below each series and antigens occuring more commonly in insulin-dependent diabetic patients are marked.

that DR3 or DR4 possessors seem to have slightly different types of diabetes (but both insulin-dependent). If these two antigens are inherited the risk is additive.

We must be careful with this concept of relative risk. The possession of two of the risk antigens may make someone more susceptible to the development of diabetes but does not imply any degree of certainty that the disease will develop. There are many people walking around who possess risk antigens in their genetic make-up but do not have diabetes and might never get it. We thus arrive at the point that there is some susceptibility to the development of diabetes in a person's genetic make-up but for the clinical development of the disease a further trigger is needed.

Studies in identical twins have been most useful in this respect. Identical twins, of course, originate in one fertilised ovum and therefore have identical genetic make-up. Thus if one twin develops diabetes but the other does not the diabetes cannot be dependent solely upon genetic make-up.

Extensive studies of diabetes in identical twins have been performed at King's College Hospital, London by Dr David Pyke and his colleagues. They have found that for insulin-dependent diabetes it is not unusual for one twin to have the disorder and the other one not. Roughly half of their twin pairs are concordant (i.e. both have insulin-dependent diabetes) and half are discordant (i.e. only one twin has diabetes). This difference must be due to environmental factors. We should add that it is not surprising that half of the twin pairs are concordant since identical twins not only have identical genetic make-up but do, to a large extent, share the same environment.

Environmental factors. For a number of years the most likely candidate for an environmental factor triggering the development of diabetes has been considered to be a viral infection. Evidence for viruses in the causation of diabetes is circumstantial. Firstly, in the six months before diabetes is diagnosed viral infections are commoner in children developing diabetes than those who do not. In particular, mumps occurs twice as often as would be predicted. Similarly, influenza has been found to be twice as common also. Secondly, in children developing diabetes there is a seasonal incidence—more children are diagnosed in autumn and in winter. These peaks coincide with the seasonal incidence of viral infections and it has been suggested tentatively that the two may be related. Thirdly, diagnosis occurs commonly around the age of 12 and to a lesser extent at 4 to 5 years and may reflect exposure to viruses around the ages of commencing schooling or changing school.

There is evidence from animal studies that infection of animals with certain viruses can produce lesions of the insulin-secreting cell and there is one report from America of a young patient with diabetic ketoacidosis and a viral infection where isolation of the virus and inocculation into animals produced diabetes.

These suggestions provide some support for a viral agent. However, even the first association between mumps or influenza and insulin-dependent diabetes would only account for about 3 per cent of children developing the disease. In addition, although it is usually assumed that the onset of insulin-dependent diabetes can be deduced with some accuracy this may not be correct. Undoubtedly some young diabetics go through a prodromal phase of minor metabolic disturbance and diminished, but not absent, insulin secretion. In these people the development of a viral illness may be sufficient to unmask diabetes, due to an increased insulin demand which cannot be met.

We have arrived at the position where a certain genetic make-up appears to make someone susceptible to developing diabetes and given exposure to an environmental agent this may precipitate the condition.

But what is the link between the two—why should a certain genetic type suffer more dire consequences of a viral infection.

Immunity. The answer may well lie in the immune response and what determines this. Certain features of the immune response to an infection are determined by genes which are located near the HLA determinants on chromosome 6. Thus a particular genetic make-up may be limited to a specific response to a viral infection. Part of this response may be the stimulation of antibody formation.

Many endocrine diseases are associated with circulating antibodies to the endocrine organ. Hypothyroidism is a good example, when in a number of cases it follows development of anti-thyroid antibodies. Insulin-dependent diabetes is similar to other hormonal disorders. Antibodies to islet cells or fractions of the cells can be found in one-third to two-thirds of newly diagnosed insulin-dependent diabetic patients and the suggestion has been made that the presence of the antibody is a marker for insulin-dependent diabetes. Islet cell antibodies also occur in normal subjects who do not develop diabetes (4 per cent) and in diabetics who are not insulin-dependent (15 per cent).Non-diabetic subjects with high titres of thyroid antibodies may also have islet cell antibodies (20 per cent) but the high incidence in newly diagnosed insulin-dependent diabetic patients implies a role for these antibodies in the causation of the disease.

Summary. There is undoubtedly a genetic susceptibility to the development of diabetes and possession of certain histo-compatibility antigens confers an increased risk for the development of insulin-dependent diabetes. This cannot entirely explain the findings in identical twins and an environmental agent must be implicated in precipitating diabetes. Viruses are likely candidates for this role but the evidence is tenuous. The exact role played by islet cell antibodies which can be detected in the blood of a high proportion of insulin-dependent diabetic patients remains unclear. Currently our best appraisal of the situation would be that a particular HLA make-up is linked to an immune response to a viral infection which results in self-directed antibodies to insulin-secreting cells. Once formed these antibodies continue to damage the cells until sufficient damage results in insulin-dependent diabetes.

Non-insulin-dependent diabetes mellitus (NIDDM)

In contrast to insulin-dependent diabetes, non-insulin-dependent diabetes mellitus is not associated with an increased frequency of HLA antigens. This should not be taken to mean that genetic factors play no part in this type of diabetes since the major histo-compatibility system is but one small part of a person's genetic make-up. Indeed the converse is true and once again Dr David Pyke's studies in identical twins have shed considerable light on the area. We must remind ourselves of the rationale of identical twin studies. similarities between pairs of twins may be genetic, since by definition the twins have identical genetic make-up, or, since they often share the same environment, similarities may be of environmental origin. Differences, however, since the genetic make-up is the same, must be due to environmental causes as was concluded from the studies of insulin-dependent pairs. The findings in pairs of non-insulin-dependent diabetic twins are as follows. When one twin has diabetes the other twin usually has it, or will develop it. Of all the pairs who have been studied the diagnosis of the second twin as having diabetes has followed within 7 years of the diagnosis in the first twin. There do remain a few pairs with one twin diabetic and the second twin having a normal glucose tolerance test but adequate follow-up will almost certainly lead to the diagnosis in the second twin. Indeed despite the normal glucose tolerance test all the second twins show metabolic abnormalities suggestive of early diabetes. These findings are consistent with a genetic component in this type of diabetes.

This finding should not be taken to imply that environmental factors are unimportant. Despite an identical genetic make-up the twins did not develop diabetes in the majority of cases until they were more than 40 years old. Why should they at this age, or even later, develop diabetes? The determinant of this could well be a change in the environment.

The most obvious candidate for an environmental agent is the development of obesity. The twin studies do not really support obesity as the trigger for the development of diabetes but it is worth considering in the rather broader light of the majority of people seen in the diabetic clinic who have developed non-insulin-dependent diabetes. Diabetes is commoner in fat people. The proportion of newly diagnosed non-insulin-dependent diabetic patients who are obese, varies from study to study but is rarely found to be less than 40 per cent and may be as high as two-thirds. In addition it is known that for World War II when food supplies declined there was a concurrent reduction in both obesity and diabetes.

Other factors which may precipitate diabetes are illnesses or trauma. The patient is often well aware of this and will ask whether an accident *caused* the diabetes to develop. It seems more likely to have unmasked diabetes than to have caused it.

We are still left with a considerable proportion of diabetic patients who are not obese when diagnosed and for whom there is no satisfactory identification of a precipitating agent. We recall that insulin-dependent diabetes is due to insulin deficiency and if, in these patients, circulating concentrations of insulin are measured they are extremely low or undetectable. The logical step would be to ask what the findings are when we look at insulin secretion in non-insulin-dependent diabetic patients.

In obese non-insulin-dependent diabetic patients it has been amply demonstrated that more insulin is secreted than in normal weight, non-diabetic subjects. This finding of raised blood glucose despite increased insulin secretion implies that

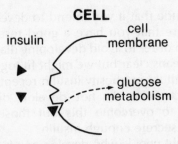

Figure 1.12 The binding of insulin to specific receptors on the cell membrane leads to its intracellular actions.

the tissues are less sensitive to insulin, or in conventional terms the subjects are insulin resistant. In recent years it has become apparent that insulin produces its effects in the cell by first binding to the cell membrane. From this binding, a train of events is set in motion which leads to metabolic action. We can go further than this since it is apparent that insulin binds at particular sites on the membrane and these sites are known as the insulin receptors (Fig. 1.12). Repeated studies have shown that obese non-insulin-dependent diabetic patients have a decreased number of receptors compared with normal subjects and thus insulin has less sites for action (Fig. 1.13)—they are insulin resistant, blood glucose rises and they are therefore diabetic.

Not all obese people have diabetes however, and if two groups of obese people are compared, a diabetic group and a normal group, the diabetic people do not secrete as much insulin as the normals. This means that compared with people of the same weight the diabetic patient secretes less insulin.

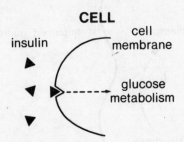

Figure 1.13 In obese non-insulin-dependent diabetic patients circulating insulin levels are raised but there is a decrease in the number of receptors on the cell membrane and a consequent impairment of intracellular actions.

We might conclude that if you intend to develop obesity you should make sure that you have a good reserve capacity to secrete insulin in order to avoid developing diabetes. This situation is by no means clear but we might fit together these two sets of findings thus: in obesity insulin receptors decrease in number: subjects who do not develop diabetes secrete enough insulin to overcome this but those who develop diabetes cannot secrete enough insulin.

In normal-weight people who develop non-insulin-dependent diabetes, insulin response to a glucose challenge is reduced. These subjects also show insulin resistance and a decreased number of insulin receptors, and the explanation of their diabetes may be similar to that of the obese subjects.

It should be added that the reduction in receptors does not fully explain the findings and a further component has been introduced. This is resistance to the action of insulin within the cell after the receptor—in jargon a 'post-receptor defect'. This is a grandiose term for something which has been known for many years. That in insulin deficiency the flow through some metabolic pathways is reduced, that is—less glucose is metabolised because some enzymes in the pathway need insulin to function efficiently.

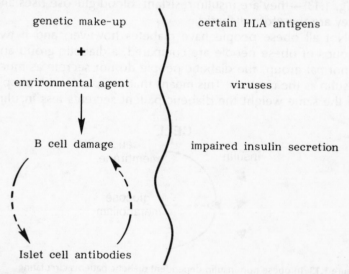

Figure 1.14 Hypothesis—the development of insulin-dependent diabetes mellitus?

Summary. To summarise the present state of knowledge of the aetiology of insulin-dependent and non-insulin-dependent diabetes, let us examine two hypotheses which are attractive. The reader should refer to the entire part of this section to assess the strength (or otherwise) of each step. Figure 1.14 puts forward a hypothesis for the development of insulin-dependent diabetes. Given an increased susceptibility to develop diabetes an environmental stimulus such as a viral infection attacks the cells which secrete insulin. Some cells are damaged and release their contents to which antibodies are formed. Given antibodies to islet cells these can now attack previously healthy cells causing further damage. When damage is sufficient insulin deficiency follows and the patient develops insulin-dependent diabetes.

Figure 1.15 suggests a hypothesis for non-insulin-dependent diabetes in obese people. Obese subjects have a decreased number of sites on cells where insulin can act and its effects are reduced. Blood glucose tends to rise and is counteracted in normal subjects by a rise in insulin returning blood glucose to normal. Those destined to get diabetes cannot increase their insulin secretion and consequently the metabolism of glucose within the cell is impaired. Hence a rise in blood glucose concentration ensues.

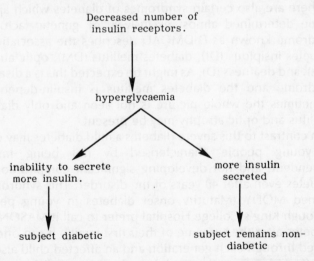

Figure 1.15 Hypothesis—the development of non-insulin-dependent diabetes mellitus?

It is interesting to note that if obese subjects successfully diet the number of insulin receptors increases. Demand for more insulin secretion is reduced and blood glucose falls—the well known results of treating obese diabetic patients by diet.

Other causes of diabetes

Having considered the two major types of diabetes we can turn to less common types.

The hormones cortisol, growth hormone, and adrenaline all have actions upon metabolism which oppose those of insulin. In disease states where excess of these hormones are secreted, diabetes may occur e.g. Cushing's syndrome, acromegaly, phaeochromocytoma.

Certain disorders which directly damage the pancreas may also result in diabetes, e.g. chronic pancreatitis, carcinoma of the pancreas, surgical removal for either of these causes, haemochromatosis with iron deposition in the pancreas.

Corticosteroid therapy may precipitate diabetes and thiazide diuretics can inhibit insulin secretion. Thiazides rarely cause diabetes but may be the final insult in someone who was just managing to meet their insulin demands. Glucose tolerance may be impaired by the contraceptive pill.

There are also certain syndromes of diabetes which appear to be determined almost exclusively by genetic factors. A syndrome known as DIDMOAD describes the association of diabetes insipidus (DI), diabetes mellitus (DM), optic atrophy (OA), and deafness (D). As might be expected this is a disabling syndrome and the diabetes mellitus is insulin-dependent. Sometimes the whole picture is not seen and only diabetes mellitus and optic atrophy may be present.

In contrast to this severe diabetes a mild diabetes may occur in young people characterised by not being insulin-dependent, and not developing significant complications of diabetes even after 40 years of the disorder. This syndrome is termed MODY (Maturity onset diabetes in young people) although King's College Hospital prefer to call it MASON type diabetes after the surname of their first family. It can often be traced through each generation and an affected child also has an affected parent. It is an interesting type of diabetes often diagnosed by oral glucose tolerance test and recognition of the syndrome may save a child from a lifetime of insulin therapy.

In comparison with insulin-dependent diabetes or non-insulin-dependent diabetes these causes of diabetes are relatively uncommon. In addition to the ones described above there are more than thirty other genetic disorders which are associated with diabetes. Unless working in a highly specialised unit most of us will not see more than one or two of these syndromes in our lifetimes.

Summary

What can go wrong?

Figure 1.16 depicts the various stages between insulin production in the B cell of the islet of Langerhans and its action within the cell.

As we have seen the predominant feature of insulin-dependent diabetes is diminished or absent insulin secretion. This step is also the major site of impairment in diabetes associated with pancreatic disease and in impaired secretion due to thiazide diuretics.

Insulin antagonists circulating in the blood include hormones with opposing actions to insulin. When insulin arrives at the cell surface it attaches to specific sites. If there are a reduced number of sites then insulin is less efficient as in non-insulin-dependent diabetes.

The effects of insulin within the cell depend upon a series of complex reactions turning, for example, glucose into energy. Some of these reactions may be sluggish and glucose metabolism is then impaired as in non-insulin-dependent diabetes.

THE NATURAL HISTORY OF DIABETES MELLITUS

In the preceding section we have dealt with current thoughts on the aetiology, and the search for a cause, of diabetes mellitus. The major sub-groups of diabetes, that is insulin-dependent and non-insulin-dependent, were considered separately since this view is supported by our present knowl-

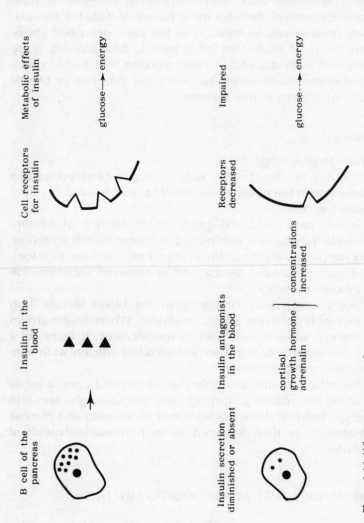

Metabolic effects of insulin

glucose ⟶ energy

Impaired

glucose ⟶ energy

Cell receptors for insulin

Receptors decreased

Insulin in the blood

Insulin antagonists in the blood

concentrations increased

cortisol
growth hormone
adrenalin

B cell of the pancreas

Insulin secretion diminished or absent

Figure 1.16 What can go wrong?

edge. It is readily apparent, however, that individual patients with diabetes of a particular type may show a widely varying course as their lives proceed with diabetes. Therefore, we must consider the natural history of the disease.

In the true meaning of the term, natural history means what happens to a patient with the disease if that patient is left untreated. Nowadays, this rarely happens since the majority of patients do not stop treatment. Nevertheless, there remains a small group of patients who default from follow-up, or manipulate their treatment, or if on diet or tablets do actually ignore dietary advice or discontinue tablets. With these few exceptions there is nothing today akin to the pre-insulin era when young people diagnosed with diabetes were likely to die within a short time. You might say that then the natural history was a death in ketoacidosis.

When discussing the natural history of diabetes today, however, both insulin-dependent and non-insulin-dependent diabetic patients have the natural history of the disease modified by treatment and this effect cannot be distinguished from the disease process itself. The extent of the impact upon the natural history of the disease which is made by successful treatment is discussed in Chapter 2, under the relationship of diabetic control to the development of complications.

In addition to the inability to separate the effect of treatment and the natural history there are certain other difficulties in any one person, be they nurse or doctor, gaining an overall impression of the course of the disease. It is not easy for those working in hospital to appreciate and keep a true perspective regarding the natural history. On the one hand, a medical ward nurse's experience can easily be limited to those patients who have gone wrong. Thus they develop a one-sided view that all diabetic patients are patients who have endless hypoglycaemic attacks, who go blind, end up with renal failure and amputated legs. On the other hand, many other nurses must wonder why so much fuss is made about asymptomatic glycosuria which is quite incidental to some other illness. The truth is that once diabetes develops it is a life-long illness with a big range of clinical effects.

It is almost true to say that once a diabetic, always a diabetic, although the severity and clinical manifestations may be related to incidental stress. It may only show during pregnancy (gestational diabetes), or when corticosteroid drugs are given. Such diabetes may be said to be 'latent' if it disappears completely when the stress is over. More often it just becomes milder and, in similar fashion, mild diabetes may become worse at times of infection and trauma, both physical and emotional. Occasionally a slight disturbance in glucose tolerance in the extremely obese may go away completely following drastic weight reduction.

In the following case histories from our clinic we would wish to make two important points. Firstly, two diabetic patients in adjacent beds or seen consecutively in the clinic may be of similar age and have been diagnosed at the same age. Despite these similarities one patient may be totally free of any long-term complications of diabetes while the next may be crippled by diabetic complications, i.e. he may be nearly blind, have had a digit or limb amputated and have heavy proteinuria. Why these two patients should differ so much is not known but emphasises the point that while we may think of the diabetic patient, he remains an individual and needs to be considered thus and followed for the rest of his life. Secondly, we can say that there is a general tendency for diabetes to get worse with time.

Illustrating the first of these points, that severe diabetes in youth can be treated effectively and be compatible with a normal useful life, our first case history deals with Anne who was born in 1930. She was admitted to a children's hospital in diabetic ketoacidosis in 1940 at the age of 10. After the initial treatment, soluble insulin was given twice a day. She had two normal pregnancies in 1952 and 1956 when the babies were induced prematurely at 36 weeks of pregnancy. In 1960 an unexpected severe 'hypo' caused a car crash. Minor background retinopathy was noticed in 1970, and now at the age of 53 she is a grandmother and works part-time. Having diabetes hardly interferes with her life except that she has to be very careful about meal times. Her retinopathy has not progressed and does not interfere with her visual acuity. Of course, there are times when she has needed expert help, and for the availability of this she has always been grateful.

There is another side to the coin, however, when in complete contrast, diabetes starting in youth can lead to fatal complications in less than twenty years. Robin was born in

Normal life

1945. At the age of 12 marked thirst and weight loss led to the diagnosis. Thereafter, he was a poor attender at school due to frequent ketoacidosis, and when finally he left school he never settled to regular work. He was always a sporadic attender in the clinic and eventually defaulted from attendance altogether. He never dieted and his insulin dose was very 'hit and miss'. Finally, he had to begin to take his diabetes seriously when in 1969 at the age of 24 he was found to have proliferative retinopathy and proteinuria. Three years later, in 1972, a foot ulcer led to below-knee amputation. In 1973, sixteen years after diagnosis and aged 28, he died from renal failure due to diabetic nephropathy, complicated by blindness due to diabetic retinopathy and the effect of widespread arterial disease. It is correct to assume that self-neglect leading to poor control of his diabetes was an important factor in causing this disaster, but, returning to our first point, it also must be admitted that there is something about the nature of 'malignant' diabetes that we do not understand. Another patient, born and developing diabetes at the same time, with a similar record of poor control and feckless behaviour, could still be alive and showing only a few signs of complications.

The second point, that diabetes gets worse in time, is illustrated by the following case history which depicts a common pattern of events. Arthur was born in 1915. He had no thoughts of diabetes until glycosuria was found at an insurance medical in 1950 when he was aged 35. At this stage his glycosuria was ignored and Arthur felt he was reprieved. After all, if his medical practitioners did not feel this a serious finding then why should Arthur think it a cause for concern? Then in 1955 glycosuria was rediscovered when he attended casualty with a carbuncle. He was advised on diet and his glycosuria disappeared. In 1960 because of persistent thirst and glycosuria, treatment with Tolbutamide was advised and this had a good effect until 1970. Now aged 55 he again had persistent glycosuria and hyperglycaemia, Metformin was added to his treatment. In 1974 at the age of 59 he had his first myocardial infarction leading to serious loss of diabetic control. Insulin treatment was necessary thereafter. Three years later in 1977, diabetic retinopathy was noted. In 1979 he had a below-knee amputation and then aged 66 he died in 1981 from a further myocardial infarction.

In this patient the disease progressed from mild and uncomplicated to severe and complicated. Although in the early years it was ignored and did not seem to matter, in the end there were serious medical problems and the disease shortened the normal expectation of life by seven years while also affecting the quality of life in his later years. We should note that although we have called the disease 'mild' in early life the problems encountered later make a rather poor joke of the term.

In general and up to now, there is about a five-fold increase in mortality compared with the general population for those who develop diabetes under the age of 10. But of course some of those dying will do so at a young age and sadly following a few years of life complicated for both them and companions by disabling diabetic complications.

So far we have only considered illustrative case histories from patients who are diagnosed at a young age. Most cases, however, are diagnosed in middle or old age (Fig. 1.17), and

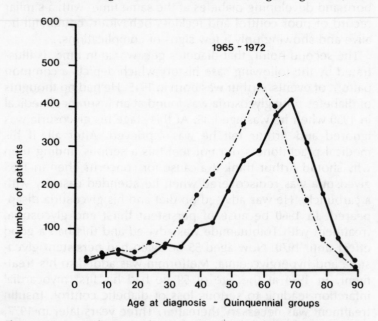

Figure 1.17 Age at diagnosis of patients attending a diabetic clinic over 5-year periods. Note the steep increase in newly diagnosed patients after the age of 45. The data cover the period 1965–1972 for both males (●--·--·--●) and females (●———●).

over the age of 50 there is about a two-fold increase in mortality. Of course, many patients who develop symptoms may have had the disease in a mild asymptomatic form for a number of years. It is important to emphasise that no-one can be quite sure when diabetes starts. The results from all mass population screening surveys have shown that for every known case of the complaint, there are half as many again who have significant diabetes needing treatment and no-one knows how long they would have escaped detection without the survey.

In addition it is not uncommon to find newly diagnosed patients presenting in middle or old age who already show the so-called long-term complications of the disease. Since we know the time taken for such complications to develop, we can safely assume that the disease has been present for more than ten to fifteen years. It was undetected, but it can hardly be thought harmless in the undiagnosed period when at diagnosis sight may be already impaired.

At the older ages, most patients are easier to manage by diet or oral treatment and in most the impact of the disease is far less. Yet this much more numerous group contains individuals who have the complaint in a severe form and who require insulin therapy—and who develop all the complications. Once again, we must emphasise that all generalisations are dangerous, that every patient must be considered individually and the nature of the disorder can change from mild to severe at any age.

So the two major sub-groups of diabetic patients, insulin-dependent and non-insulin-dependent may be distinct in terms of treatment, in terms of aetiology, and in biochemical terms. Where the groups join is in the development of complications with both groups at risk of the disabling complications which are considered further in Chapter 3. Even within a group there may be a wide variation in the course the disease runs and to date we have no good explanation of this. One insulin-dependent diabetic patient may have 'malignant' diabetes, suffering in a major way within ten years of diagnosis, while yet another may have 'mild' diabetes. In this context by 'mild' we mean that the patient is free of complications after twenty to thirty years of diabetes. We have no way of knowing which group a patient will fall into and all must receive the same degree of treatment and care and advice. It is worth repeating that 'mild' is an adjective we abhor, in most instances, to describe diabetes. Mild or severe cannot be predicted and what appears mild one year may be severe five years later. It is a term to be used by those with prophetic insight and a term to be rejected when it may induce in the patient, the nurse, and the doctor an approach to managing the disorder which may be a source of intense regret when our patient reaches later life and its problems.

In the above we have tried to portray the variability and the seriousness of diabetes mellitus. The natural history of diabetes mellitus is such that the diagnosis can never be ignored nor the disease treated lightly in a single one of our patients. If doubts remain on this score we conclude this section with some hard facts which we will return to in Chapter 3.

Compared with the normal population, diabetic patients have a two-fold increase in the incidence of myocardial infarction, a five-fold increase in gangrene, and a two-fold increase in cerebrovascular disease.

In an average diabetic clinic 20 per cent of patients will have signs of diabetic neuropathy and 10 per cent will have symptoms.

Proteinuria in diabetic men, and in diabetic women under the age of 40, is usually due to diabetic renal disease and affects somewhere around 10 per cent of clinic attenders. In diabetic patients diagnosed under the age of 20 years, half of them die from renal disease.

Between the ages of 30 to 64, diabetic retinopathy is the single most common cause of blindness in England and Wales.

2

Diagnosis and treatment of diabetes

DIAGNOSIS OF DIABETES

Diagnosis is important

Correct diagnosis is always important. Never more so than in a life-long complaint like diabetes mellitus. All population surveys have shown that undiagnosed and therefore neglected, florid diabetes is common. On the other hand, it is quite wrong to over-diagnose the complaint and inflict need-less restrictions and fear on those who are merely under sus-picion. It is well to remember the penalty of being called diabetic for life assurance or employment purposes. We must admit there is a difficult borderline between what we call normal and abnormal.

Diabetic symptoms

Diagnosis is easy in patients with acute and classical symptoms such as thirst, polyuria and weakness. Insidious weight loss is an important sign of diabetes but unfortunately in the figure conscious, weight loss is often a cause for self-congratulation and is attributed to the good effects of the latest diet. It is well known that pruritus vulvae is an important symptom of diabetes. It is less well understood that there is a male counter part of balanitis, and circumcision is definitely not the first treatment of choice if there is glycosuria! So much glucose may be present in diabetic urine that it can show as white deposits from dried out splashes of urine on shoes and underclothes.

On the other hand, significant diabetes may be quite asymptomatic and only come to light as the result of a routine urine test in the out-patients department or during a medical for a job. Often, such patients who may deny any symptoms still feel much better for treatment.

Patients with previously undiagnosed diabetes often present to the optician or the eye clinic. This is because blurred vision may result from changes in refraction due to hyperglycaemia, cataract formation, or diabetic retinopathy. In the latter case we must presume that the diabetes has been present for many years. Similarly, patients with unsuspected diabetes may present to the chiropodist, the orthopaedic clinic, or casualty department because of neuropathic foot ulcers. The neurologist may be asked to see patients with foot drop or neuritic pain and again unsuspected diabetes may be the underlying cause. The polyuria of untreated diabetes may aggravate the symptoms of prostatism, while peripheral arterial disease causing intermittent claudication or gangrene may take the patient to a vascular surgeon. Furuncles, carbuncles and necrobiosis may lead to the patient attending a dermatologist.

Such presentations demand that nurses and doctors retain a high index of suspicion of diabetes. We would do well to remember that so-called 'routine' urine testing has only become routine because it is held to be of importance. In many patients, correct diagnosis and hence treatment has only come about because the practice nurse, the nurse in out-patients, or the ward nurse remembered to test the urine.

Urine testing

The essential routine to establish the correct diagnosis is still to do a urine test and consider the result. The best specimen to test is the one passed after a meal. If glycosuria is also present in the fasting specimen it is even more significant, but on the other hand, the milder forms of diabetes can be missed.

Reagents for urine testing

Clinistix (Ames) is an enzyme impregnated strip that detects glucose only, and is useful for screening. Unfortunately, to help overcome the effect of occasional inhibitors found in normal urine and in patients taking certain drugs, it has to be made very sensitive and may sometimes give misleadingly positive results because of minute amounts of glucose which can be present in normal urine. Diastix (Ames) like Clinistix is also based on a specific glucose enzyme but the colour reaction is different. The reaction must be read at 30 seconds after dipping the paper for 2 seconds. It can record up to 2 per cent glycosuria. A weakness is that the brown colour development may be retarded by a high concentration of ketones. A simultaneous ketone test will avoid this difficulty. Another important source of error for both Diastix and Ketostix is that they do not work if either the urine or the reagent strips are at refrigeration temperature. The bottles should be stored in a dark dry place and well stoppered after use and it must be remembered that the strips deteriorate and should not be used after the expiry date.

Boehringer (Mannheim) have recently introduced an improved enzyme urine testing strip called Diabur Test 5000. It has a double panel of colours like the 20:800 blood testing strip which extends the range of the test from 0.1 per cent to 5 per cent. It is not upset by ketones but has the disadvantage that it has to be read at two minutes.

Clinitest Reagent tablets (Ames) depend on an entirely different principle. They are a convenient adaptation of the old Fehlings and Benedicts test. The tablets contain copper sulphate, sodium hydroxide, sodium carbonate and citric acid. When added to urine and water they effervesce and generate heat. In the alkaline medium, glucose reduces the blue copper sulphate solution to reddish insoluble cuprous oxide. The final colour of the mixture indicates the proportion of sugar in the mixture up to 2 per cent. The test must be done exactly as recommended otherwise it will give misleading results. The tablets deteriorate rapidly if exposed to air. They are very corrosive if swallowed and can cause serious oesophageal burns and subsequent stricture, so advice to the parents of young children on how and where to store the tablets is important.

Blood testing

If our patient has diabetic symptoms and heavy glycosuria in excess of 1 per cent, then the diagnosis of diabetes mellitus is extremely likely. It always needs confirming by measuring the blood glucose concentration. As with urine, this is better done after a normal breakfast or lunch and tests done fasting or a long time after the preceding meal can be misleading. In any case the time and nature of the last meal is worth recording. Diagnosis is so important that the initial blood test should be carried out by a laboratory subject to quality control analysis. Above all, the result should be recorded for posterity so it is possible to recall the blood glucose figure years later. In a patient with symptoms and glycosuria, a post-prandial blood glucose of 11.0 mmol/l or more establishes the diagnosis. Similarly, a fasting level in excess of 8.0 mmol/l is always abnormal. In cases of doubt it is always worthwhile repeating the test. Blood may be taken by venepuncture or by pricking the finger or ear lobe (capillary). There are small differences between the two in the post-absorptive state. If a venous sample has to be stored before analysis it is important that the container has some fluoride to act as a glucose preservative. Capillary specimens can also be sent to the laboratory in fine tubes or read from an ingenious method using a drop of blood spotted on to filter paper.

The careful screening and measurement of blood glucose lead to confirmation of the diagnosis of diabetes mellitus in about 80 per cent of patients who find their way to the diabetic clinic. When results are equivocal, however, a glucose tolerance test may be necessary.

Glucose tolerance tests

The glucose tolerance test is not often required to confirm a diagnosis of clinical diabetes and its main use is to exclude diabetes, to sort out the non-diabetic causes of glycosuria and to establish the diagnosis of a very mild diabetic state when it is important as in pregnancy and in youth. The patient is fasted overnight and a blood and urine sample obtained before 75 g of diluted glucose is drunk. Blood is then taken at 30 minute intervals and urine at hourly intervals for 2 or 2½ hours. Up to the test the patient should eat normally and during the test the patient should sit quietly and not smoke. Timing has to be accurate and the blood glucose has to be measured using a full laboratory method rather than the useful but somewhat inaccurate methods in common use on the wards or in the diabetic clinic. We do not propose to deal with all the minutae of the arbitrary distinctions between normal and abnormal. It is important to state, however, that minor degrees of 'abnormality' become increasingly common with advancing age when they matter least.

In Figure 2.1 all the blood glucose measurements are abnormal and we can say that the test was unnecessary. Certainly the fasting measurement was grossly abnormal and should have clinched the diagnosis. It is also likely that a sample taken after a meal would have been abnormal and we must conclude that the test was requested from ignorance. The only thing we can say in favour of the test was that the multiple analyses made the diagnosis certain.

This unnecessary requesting of the oral glucose tolerance test is far from uncommon and is a considerable waste of

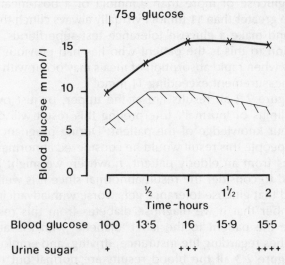

Blood glucose	10·0	13·5	16	15·9	15·5
Urine sugar	+		+++		++++

Figure 2.1 Blood glucose and urine tests during an oral glucose tolerance test. Glucose was drunk after a fasting blood and urine specimen were taken. All the blood measurements were abnormal and increasing glycosuria during the test was found. The upper limit of the normal range for blood glucose is marked (⊤⊤⊤⊤)

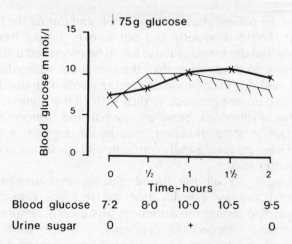

Figure 2.2 Blood glucose and urine tests during an oral glucose tolerance test. Glucose was drunk after a fasting blood and urine specimen were taken. The results are all at, or above, the upper limit of the normal range (▽▽▽▽)

laboratory resources. Once again we would stress that a fasting blood glucose of more than 8 mmol/l or a post-meal blood glucose greater than 11 mmol/l virtually always clinch the diagnosis and make a glucose tolerance test superfluous. A rare exception to this is the patient who has had previous gastric surgery when rapid absorption of meals may occur with a post-meal measurement exceeding 11 mmol/l.

In Figure 2.2 all results are at the upper, or just over the upper limits of 'normal'. Interpreting this result will depend upon our knowledge of the patient. During pregnancy or in young people this result would be considered abnormal. If the test was from an elderly patient, however, we might be less inclined to consider the result abnormal since it is well documented that glucose tolerance gets worse with advancing age. Remember that if we diagnose diabetes from this result we confine the patient to the label 'diabetic' with the attached difficulties regarding life insurance, driving, and employment.

In Figure 2.3 all the blood results are normal but there is glycosuria throughout the test. This result is uncommon and of no real clinical importance. It indicates the condition of renal glycosuria—the spillage of glucose into the urine at blood levels not normally associated with glycosuria. Here the

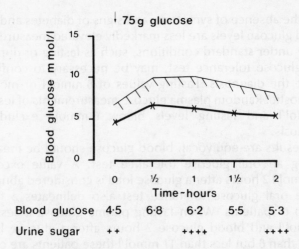

| Blood glucose | 4·5 | 6·8 | 6·2 | 5·5 | 5·3 |
| Urine sugar | ++ | | ++++ | ++++ | |

Figure 2.3 Results from a glucose tolerance test showing renal glycosuria. All the blood results are lower than the upper limit of the normal range ($\overline{\wedge\wedge\wedge\wedge}$) but throughout the test the patient had glycosuria

blood results are important in excluding the diagnosis of diabetes. An important point here is that the patient needs a clear explanation of the finding or, better, a copy of the test result since it is likely that glycosuria will be encountered at medical examinations throughout the patient's life. Clear appreciation of the finding may save the patient from repeated trips to a diabetic clinic and glucose tolerance tests.

Criteria for diagnosis

Recently the World Health Organization and the National Diabetes Data Group in America have published revised criteria for the diagnosis of diabetes. Unfortunately there are small differences between the two sets of criteria underlining the difficulties of separating normal and abnormal.

The W.H.O. criteria, which are likely to find wide acceptance in Europe, state that in the presence of symptoms such as severe thirst, increased urine and glycosuria, and rapid weight loss, the diagnosis is simply confirmed by a random plasma glucose concentration which exceeds 11 mmol/l. Alternatively the presence of specific microvascular disease, usually retinopathy, also establishes the diagnosis.

In the absence of symptoms and signs of diabetes and when blood glucose levels are less markedly elevated measurements made under standard conditions, such as fasting or during an oral glucose tolerance test, may be necessary to confirm or refute the diagnosis. Fasting values of 8 mmol/l or more are diagnostic. Random plasma glucose measurements of less than 8 mmol/l and fasting levels bleow 6 mmol/l exclude the diagnosis.

If results are equivocal, blood glucose should be measured during an oral glucose tolerance test. A value exceeding 11 mmol/l 2 hours after a glucose load is considered abnormal.

The oral glucose tolerance test also delineates a further group of patients. When fasting plasma glucose is less than 8 mmol/l and blood glucose 2 hours after a glucose load is more than 8 but less than 11 mmol/l these patients are considered to have 'impaired glucose tolerance'. It should be noted that using older criteria for the diagnosis of diabetes many of these patients would be considered diabetic. The new category has been introduced following a number of epidemiological studies. The findings in these studies indicate that subjects with 2 hour glucose values within this range rarely show development of the specific complications of diabetes (particularly microangiopathy). In addition only a small proportion show worsening to diabetes. These findings might lead us to conclude that such subjects should be considered normal. Unfortunately, within this group there is an increased frequency of macrovascular disease. This is increased compared with normal subjects but does not reach the levels associated with diabetes. Nevertheless we must consider such patients to be at risk of disease of large arteries.

A practical point which has not been completely resolved is what we tell the patient with this variety of oral glucose tolerance test. In general, patients attend a diabetic clinic initially to learn whether or not they have diabetes. We can tell them that for purposes of life insurance, or employment they do not have diabetes. We cannot say with any conviction, however, that they are normal since we appreciate that such subjects fall into an at-risk group for macrovascular complications. To the patient this may be a source of confusion.

A further unresolved point is whether such patients should be subjected to repeated follow-up in the diabetic clinic. It may well be that this will vary from clinic to clinic but at present we continue to see such patients in the clinic from time to time.

DIET

Introduction

It is part of folklore that anyone diagnosed as being diabetic should have a diet and newly diagnosed patients do not feel they have been properly looked after unless they have a booklet with do's and don'ts about what they should or should not eat. Whether they get good professional advice or not, they are all too ready to supplement this with bad advice from diabetic friends who have always eaten 'just what they fancied' or suffer the attentions of well-meaning relatives who will press unsuitable food with such words as 'a little bit of cake will not do you any harm just this once' (Fig. 2.4). Eating is a very basic human activity. Meal times are the simplest and the most enduring human pleasure and an important daily ceremony of family life. It follows that any advice to alter the pattern of everyday eating must be given with care and due regard to the individual.

Nurse or dietician?

We feel that the nurse expert in diabetes must be prepared to talk to her patient about food and know about theories and fashions in dietetics. In this they must not feel they are in conflict with the dietician. The basic pattern of the diet is often laid out by the dietician. Advice given at a single interview, however, often at the end of an exhausting first visit to a hospital clinic, cannot be expected to impart enough knowledge to last a lifetime. Intelligent and inquisitive patients will read about the subject and simple questions may then arise which the nurse must be expected to consider. The less intelligent, the sick, and the emotionally disturbed patient will not take in anything following the first interview and it should then fall to the nurse with close contact and knowledge of the individual patient to get across the essential information. The dietician's role remains that of the expert in food who can be consulted.

History

Before the advent of insulin in 1923, a doctor's advice was the only treatment for diabetes. John Rollo (1797) may be regarded as the pioneer of modern dieting treatment and his observation that this was effective was confirmed by many others. The French physician, Appollinaire Bouchardat (1806–86) noticed the beneficial effects of privation on his diabetic patients during the seige of Paris in 1870. He invented the slogan, which is still excellent advice, 'Manger les moins possible' (Eat the least possible). He tried to fit the diet to the individual patient and was the first to emphasise the value of exercise. The practice of undernutrition was carried to the extreme limit in the U.S.A. by F.M. Allen (1919) who was able to extend the life expectancy of diabetic children from 1.3 to 2.9 years by restricting calories severely and reducing carbohydrate to 30 g or in some cases even as low as 5 g a day. Since the introduction of insulin there has been a gradual relaxation but, as in the past, there have been advocates for every permutation of the proportions of protein, carbohydrate and fat. In recent times, emphasis has been given both to the possibility of limiting vascular disease by reducing fat intake, and by the substitution of polyunsaturated for saturated fat, as well as by using dietary fibre to slow the rate of absorption of sugar.

Sugar

The simplest and most non-controversial dietetic advice to the diabetic patient is to do without sugar.

The abnormal increase of the blood glucose in even the mildest diabetic patients to the 75 g of pure glucose which we give in the standard glucose tolerance test, shows that by definition the diabetic patient cannot adapt quickly to refined sugar because of its rapid absorption from the bowel. A similar response is found to sucrose (cane or beet sugar) and honey. There will be an immediate improvement in diabetic symptoms and a reduction in the level of hyperglycaemia in all sorts of diabetic patients by simply doing without sugar. Remember, before diagnosis the patient may well have increased sugar consumption by drinking 'pop' or other sweetened drinks in response to the thirst of uncontrolled diabetes. In any case,

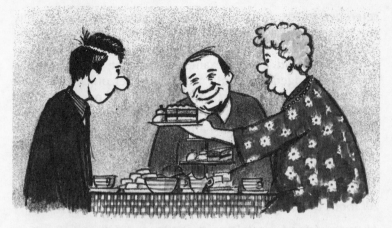

'A LITTLE BIT OF CAKE WILL DO YOU NO HARM JUST THIS ONCE'

Figure 2.4 'Temptation'

the average national consumption of sugar is very high and in some it may provide a significant proportion of the total calorie intake. Consider the not unusual case of the patient who drinks 10 cups of sweetened tea a day. Two teaspoonfuls of sugar is 10 g of carbohydrate and hence 100 g of carbohydrate is 410 cal and this could be 25 per cent of the total daily intake. Confectionery containing a large proportion of sugar is widely advertised as a desirable source of quick energy. Sugar is a cheap ingredient used to improve the taste of a whole range of processed foods. Yet the nurse can remind her patient that it is not a necessary item of diet and refining is only an invention of the last 200 years. Thus, good initial advice to *all* diabetic patients is to cut out completely sugar, glucose, jam, marmalade, honey, syrup, sweets, chocolates, treacle, buns, cakes, sweet biscuits, chocolate biscuits, pastry, tinned fruit, pop, lucozade, ribena and sweet wines.

The obese diabetic patient

Restriction of all types of food intake is the key to successful treatment for those who carry an excess proportion of fat. Desirable weight for new patients should be worked out with reference to sex, height and age, and very significant obesity can then be defined as those in excess of 20 per cent of the ideal body weight. In practice some account needs to be taken of the body build, and for example a thick set, muscular frame should be judged differently from a slender office worker. A way round this difficulty is to measure the thickness of the fold of skin and subcutaneous fat which can be pinched up where it is loose over the trunk and arms. In practice, the trained eye can soon pick out the truly obese from those of heavy, muscular build.

All foods are interconvertible

All type of food, protein, carbohydrate or fat after digestion and absorption, is broken down to a few relatively simple substances which can then be recombined to build up new tissue or used as a fuel. It follows that anything taken in excess of day to day requirements can be used to build up fatty tissue.

Some foods are much more concentrated than others. Table 2.1 lists some common high calorific value foods. They usually contain a large proportion of fat, or are concentrated 'convenience' foods. Conversely all vegetables and fruits are of low calorific value (Table 2.2) and good general advice is to follow Candide's advice and at the same time gain the additional benefit of healthy exercise 'Mais il faut cultiver notre jardin' (But we must cultivate our garden). A most useful reference

Table 2.1 Examples of high calorific value foods in a form prepared for eating.

	Cal/100 g(/3.5 oz)
Cheese (Cheddar)	406
Butter	740
Cream (double)	447
Sausage (grilled)	318
Salted peanuts	570
Potato crisps	533
Chips	253
Pork pie	376
Salami	491
Whisky	222

Table 2.2 Examples of low calorific value foods in a form prepared for eating.

	Cal/100 g(/3.5 oz)
Boiled potatoes	80
Apple (weighed with skin and core)	35
Cabbage (boiled spring)	7
Runner beans	19
Leeks	24
Lettuce	12
Poached fish	94
Carrots	19
Wine (Dry)	68
Porridge	44

book is *McCance and Widdowson's, The Composition of Foods*, HMSO, London, 4th edition, 1978.

As is well known, the main problem of getting the obese diabetic patient to eat less is a psychological one. Most obese people dislike being fat, dislike talking about it and have developed complex mechanisms for avoiding a confrontation with their obesity. Often they have become discouraged by failure after trying the various dieting methods widely advocated in books and magazines. Patients often feel that life is unfair. Unfortunately, the relationship between food intake and energy expenditure is very complex and there is now good evidence to show that those who stay thin in spite of eating well, do so because they can burn off excess calories. Many obese women do not eat excessively—overweight men are more likely to be gross feeders. Nevertheless, the principle holds good for both sexes that the obese diabetic patient needs to lose weight in order to achieve good diabetic control and this can only be done by eating less. It is our ability to persuade the patient that dieting is worthwhile that counts. Having diabetes is often considered by patients a powerful reason for taking advice seriously and some patients can surprise us by doing exactly what they are told. They all deserve the benefit of being properly instructed once. Very mild diabetes in the very obese can go into lasting remission following considerable and sustained weight reduction and this is the one form of the complaint for which it is possible to claim a 'cure'.

Diet for the normal weight diabetic patient

Our ideas about the proper advice for the lean and healthy patient whether they are on insulin, tablets or just diet alone, has undergone considerable change in recent years. We no longer believe that carbohydrate restriction other than doing without simple sugar is correct. The advice to eat ordinary or even generous amounts of wholemeal bread, potatoes, and other starchy foods, is against the accepted beliefs of most patients with longstanding diabetes and most doctors and nurses, who are slightly behind the times.

As an example we can take Leonard Thompson who was the first patient ever to receive insulin in 1922 in Toronto. He was advised to take the sort of diet which became customary for many years which we now consider excessively high in fats. Table 2.3 compares the percent of total calorie intake derived from protein, fat and carbohydrate in the Thompson diet with the average American diet and what is now considered desirable for the general and diabetic populations of the U.S.A.

Numerous studies have now shown that diets which are rich in complex carbohydrates (starch) and fibre not only allow for good blood glucose control, but also markedly reduce serum cholesterol and triglycerides. Diets that contain large amounts of fat are well known to be 'atherogenic' at least in susceptible persons. In other words, the diet best for diabetic patients is no different from the one recommended for general health. The customary diet in Japan and other Eastern countries has traditionally been high carbohydrate/low fat and up to now it is known that in these countries coronary artery disease , even in diabetic patients, is uncommon.

Table 2.3 Percentage of calories derived from food sources in different diets

Nutrient	'Thomson' diet	'Average' American diet	Dietary 'goals' for U.S. citizens	American Diabetes Association Recommendation
		Percent of total calorie intake		
Protein	9.8	12	12	12–20
Fat	70.6	42	30	20–38
Carbohydrate	19.6	48	58	50–60

Exchanges

All this is not to say that the well-informed diabetic patient does not need to know about 10 g exchanges, rations or portions of carbohydrate. The crux of the matter is, that the patient on insulin needs equivalent amounts of carbohydrate at approximately the same times every day to balance the hypoglycaemic effect of the injected insulin. Thus, both the timing and distribution of the carbohydrate needs to be considered. We should also take into account the amount and pattern of physical activity. Hypoglycaemia from unbalanced insulin action can be a very serious problem if there is too long an interval between meals; so meals need to be at least five hourly and it is important not to forget the bed-time snack for fear of nocturnal hypoglycaemia. If the patient understands the system of 10 g exchanges it allows for variety in meals and gets round the problem of eating away from home. A list of exchanges is given in Appendix 1. The weights referred to are cooked unless otherwise stated. Each 10 g exchange is 41 cal.

The perfect patient

Let us take an extreme example of a careful, intelligent, well-motivated and well set-up patient.

James Smith   Male   Aged 35 years

Sedentary work, but golf and gardening Saturdays and Sundays, Wife cooks.

Weight 70 kg (11 stone)   Height 183 cm (6 ft)

His per cent ideal body weight is 100 per cent and therefore his present calorie intake is well balanced with his needs. Treatment is with a mixture of Soluble and Isophane twice daily. Dietary history suggests a daily weekday intake of 1800 cal—more at weekends.

We have already suggested that 55 per cent of total calories should be carbohydrate (Table 2.3) = 990 Calories

Divide by 41 to convert to 10 g exchanges

$$\frac{990}{41} = 24 \text{ exchanges}$$

Distribution as follows:

Breakfast   any 5 from list

Lunch   any 7 from list

Tea   any 2 from list
Dinner   any 8 from list
Last thing   any 2 from list

For weekend extra activity add 2R to breakfast and 2R for mid-morning snack.

This recommended diet will probably differ from the accustomed intake. This is because the advice to cut out refined sugar and to increase the proportion of carbohydrate from 48 to 55 per cent will mean an increased intake of starchy food. If the calorie intake is to remain constant there will also need to be a reduction of fat intake by a small amount from 81 g to 59 g (about 1 oz of butter). There should be *no* need to change the amount of meat, fish, eggs, cheese, fresh green vegetables and certain fruits *normally* eaten since the patient is not overweight.

The virtues of fibre

Dietary fibre is important in the diabetic diet. Carbohydrate from foodstuffs rich in fibre is more slowly absorbed from the bowel and this reduces the sudden post-meal rise in blood glucose which is always a difficulty for diabetic patients. Fibre is the supporting framework of the plant cell wall which is resistant to the digestive juices and has no nutritional value. It does provide bulk to the stool and is very helpful in avoiding constipation. Unfortunately, the modern milling of wheat grain removes all fibre. Our patients should be encouraged to eat wholemeal bread, porridge oats, beans and fresh unprocessed fruit and vegetables. They can add unsweetened bran. This would be sound general advice for all types of patients whether diabetic or not.

Unsaturated fats?

We have already suggested that because of the great importance of ischaemic heart and leg disease, the ideal diabetic diet should not become too rich in fat. The next question is whether all fats are the same. The solid fats of animal origin such as those found in milk, cream, butter, cheese and meat consist mainly of so-called saturated fatty acids. It is believed that these increase plasma cholesterol, whereas the fatty acids of the unsaturated type found in corn and sunflower oil, fish and many nuts do the reverse and actually lower plasma cholesterol concentration. Bacon fat and olive oil are neutral and have little effect either way. In practice, we must be careful not to deprive our patients of too many of the good things of life. It is our practice to counsel moderation in the use of butter, cream and cheese and use corn oil for cooking.

Patient compliance

It will come as no surprise to nurses that many of our patients are unwilling or incapable of following any complicated dietetic instruction. We should have few illusions. Thirty years ago, there was a careful enquiry about dietary knowledge and practice in 94 established diabetic patients attending Leeds General Infirmary. Only 16 were considered satisfactory. Forty-four showed moderate knowledge but 34 were quite hopeless. There is no reason to believe there has been any great change today. Some are willing to follow advice for a short time but then give up. The elderly are not prepared to change the habits of a lifetime. Sometimes an unrealistic diet is prescribed which takes no account of the needs of hard physical work. A powerful and understandable reason for those on insulin is fear of hypoglycaemic attacks. Some are unaccustomed to a set pattern of meal times and others have no understanding of the basic terms such as protein, fat or carbohydrate.

Simple instruction

This being so, there is much to be said for keeping dietary advice very simple. Thus, a mild case who is overweight can be instructed to 'keep off sugar and sweet things. Use artificial sweeteners. Only take small helpings of your usual food and do not eat between meals. Avoid fried food, chips and crisps. Test your urine if you think you have eaten the wrong thing.'For those on insulin. 'Eat no sugar or anything with sugar in it. Enjoy your usual helping of all other kinds of food, but keep to the same meal times and try to eat much the same amount from day to day. Eat more if you have more exercise. Always have a bed-time snack and do not miss a meal'.

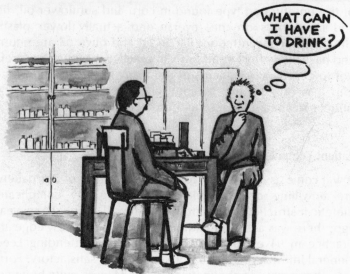

WHAT CAN I HAVE TO DRINK?

Figure 2.5 'Prohibition?'

Alcohol

The topic of drink is often uppermost in the patient's mind when treatment is first discussed. There is the unspoken fear of a medical instruction for total prohibition! (Fig. 2.5). Spirits are unsuitable for the obese since every 50 ml of whisky or gin contains 100 cal, but they contain no sugar. A pint of beer contains about 20 g of carbohydrate (2 exchanges) as well as the alcohol and altogether this yields about 250 cal. It is, therefore, also unsuitable for weight reduction but can be fitted in to the standard diet provided it is not taken to excess. Wine, although expensive, is the most suitable drink. Unless sweet, it only contains about 1 g of carbohydrate per bottle and has only between 2 or 3 times the alcohol strength of beer. Alcohol may cause facial flushing in some patients taking sulphonylureas (p. 73). It may also be a factor in causing hypoglycaemic attacks since in excess it may reduce glucose production by the liver. In general, however, moderate amounts of alcohol are quite suitable for most patients with diabetes.

Diet in illness

What to eat in illness and other emergencies is always a matter for concern to patients and often their relatives. For mild cases on diet alone there should be no difficulty and general advice to drink plenty of fluids, artificially sweetened if desired, and to live on soup, toast and milk is usually appropriate. This is also correct for patients on tablets except that it is important to guard against hypoglycaemia by advising them to take some form of carbohydrate at least every eight hours. Metformin therapy should not be continued if there is an upset stomach or diarrhoea (p. 77). There are circumstances when sulphon-ylurea therapy can be temporarily discontinued if the patient is not eating anything but it is vital to check that the urine remains sugar-free and the blood glucose normal. More often intercurrent illness, particularly infection and recumbency, makes diabetes worse and there may be an indication for temporary insulin therapy (Ch. 6). Patients on insulin present the greatest problem. If they cannot tolerate solid food at the usual meal times their usual carbohydrate exchanges will need making up with some sweet palatable fluid. A pint of milk with 5 g of Ovaltine or Horlicks is 40 g (4 exchanges). The urine will need testing for glucose and ketones and the type and dose of insulin may need changing.

Children

Diabetic children need properly prepared, well-balanced food at regular meal times. Somehow they need protection from their friends, relatives and the bandishments of the confec-tionery industry so as not to associate a treat with eating sweets or chocolate. Obesity can be a great problem in adolescent girls (Ch. 6). It is important to ensure they are not being over-dosed with insulin and that the diet has not become too rich in fats.

Unusual activity

This is an important problem for the insulin-treated patient and is a potent cause of hypoglycaemic attacks (Ch. 6). For strenu-ous team games and athletics, confectionery taken before the exertion and at halftime is justified. How much to take, has to be left to trial and error and the patient's good sense. It is also important to advise extra carbohydrate food for the next meal after the activity since hypoglycaemia can be a delayed effect. In general it is better to anticipate extra physical activity by eating bigger ordinary meals in advance of, and during the activity, than waiting to put things right with sugar or sweets when trouble starts.

Non-European diets

The traditional Indian diet based on chapati or rice, rich in vegetables and low in fat has a high proportion of carbohydrate and fibre. We have already suggested that, contrary to popular belief and *provided* the patient is not obese , this is very suitable for diabetes. The difficulty comes when overeating and inactivity cause obesity, and in these circumstances the only realistic and often fruitless instruction is to eat less. Fasting for religious reasons needs consideration and during the Moslem month of Ramadan when nothing is eaten during daylight the timing of insulin or tablet treatment needs altering to coincide with the first meal taken after sunset.

Special diabetic foods

Special foods for diabetic patients are widely advertised but do not find much favour. Some contain sorbitol which, although sweet, is not well absorbed and may provoke diarrhoea. Some are sweetened with fructose which is similar to glucose and needs counting in the diet. The best for those who are fond of them and can make do in small amounts are the marmalade and jam.

The British Diabetic Association recommends that fructose be used by diabetic patients without consideration of its carbohydrate value so long as their total intake in any one day does not exceed 50 g in weight. Fructose is not low in calories, however, and must not be used in any form by those diabetic patients who are having to control their calorie intake. We recommend that special foods where fructose is present should not have the carbohydrate value of that fructose counted, as long as the 50 g maximum/day has not been exceeded. For example, if a chocolate bar contains 30 g carbohydrate (of which 15 g is fructose) then that bar need only be counted as 15 g not 30 g.

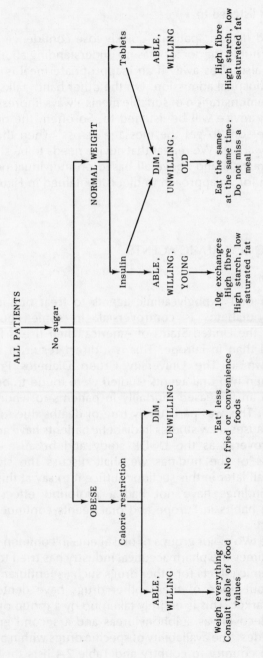

Figure 2.6 A synopsis of the tactics for dietary advice to diabetic patients

The nurse is listened to

Experienced diabetic patients quickly lose confidence if they sense their nurse (or doctor) has no understanding about their diet. Trust also ebbs away if an inappropriate meal is served soon after hospital admission. On the other hand, talks about food and demonstration of suitable meals always impresses the patient and advice will be listened to. So often, the nurse is the only person 'to get the message across' when the right opportunity arises. We repeat that advice needs to be straight-forward, practical and above all based on individual need. A simple plan for an approach to diet is contained in Figure 2.6.

ORAL HYPOGLYCAEMIC AGENTS

Introduction

The use of oral hypoglycaemic agents to treat non-insulin-dependent diabetes is controversial. In some countries, particularly the United States of America, their use is far less widespread than in Europe. This is a direct result of a large study known as The University Group Diabetes Program (UGDP) when two oral agents studied were found to be asso-ciated with an increased mortality in patients to whom they were given. This was particularly true of deaths due to cardi-ovascular causes. Few studies in diabetic patients have aroused such controversy as the UGDP study and because of the implications of the findings we shall discuss the study in greater detail later in this section. Suffice it to say at this time, that the findings have not had a profound effect upon prescribing habits in Europe and oral agents continue to be widely used.

There are two major groups of oral agents in common usage. At various times the pharmaceutical industry has tried to claim hypoglycaemic effects for other drugs such as fenfluramine or clofibrate but none of these other drugs have dented the lucrative market. This is entirely taken up by a group of drugs known collectively as sulphonylureas and a second group— the biguanides. The availability of specific drugs within a group varies from country to country and Table 2.4 lists the drugs.

Table 2.4 Oral hypoglycaemic agents

Sulphonylureas	*Trade names*
Chlorpropamide	Diabenese, Melitase, Glymese
Glibenclamide	Daonil, Semi-daonil, Euglucon
Glibornuride	Glutril
Gliclazide	Diamicron
Glipizide	Glibenese, Minodiab
Gliquidone	Glurenorm
Tolazamide	Tolanase
Tolbutamide	Rastinon, Pramidex
Sulphonylurea-related	
Acetohexamide	Dimelor
Glymidine	Gondafon
Biguanides	
Buformin	(i)
Metformin	Glucophage
Phenformin	(ii)

(i) not available in U.K.
(ii) not routinely available in U.K.

The hypoglycaemic effect of both groups of drugs were accidental findings. Hypoglycaemia occurring during sulphonamide treatment of typhoid fever led to the recognition of sulphonylureas as hypoglycaemic agents, while hypoglycaemia following removal of the parathyroids in animals was attributed to guanidine and led to the development of biguanides—guanidine derivatives.

Sulphonylureas

How do they work?

Sulphonylureas have been used to treat non-insulin-dependent diabetic patients for approximately 25 years and yet despite this, the mechanism of action remains unclear. In part this is due to uncertainty of the basic defect in non-insulin-dependent diabetes which was discussed in Chapter 1.

It is clear that in the short term, ingestion of a sulphonylurea increases insulin secretion from the B cell of the islets of Langerhans. This occurs if sulphonylureas are given to animals, normal subjects, or diabetic patients with the ability to secrete some insulin. It does not occur when sulphonylureas are given to animals following destruction of the B cells, or in insulin-

dependent diabetic patients who produce no insulin. Sulphonylureas therefore, only work in patients who have some
secretion of insulin.

During long term administration, however, the picture
becomes more confused since the hypoglycaemic effects
persist but the insulin-stimulating ability appears to be lost.

An example of this is an excellent study carried out in
America. Non-insulin-dependent diabetic patients were given
a baseline oral glucose tolerance test and glucose and insulin
responses were measured. Not surprisingly, since they were
diabetic, blood glucose was raised and serum insulin
responses were impaired. The patients were then given glibenclamide for six months and glucose tolerance tests were
repeated at 2 and at 6 months. At 2 months there was a marked
improvement in the insulin response and consequently a more
normal glucose response, demonstrating the short term effect
of the sulphonylurea upon insulin secretion. After six months,
however, the insulin response had returned to that obtained
in the baseline study. Instead of a deterioration in blood
glucose response to baseline values, it remained at the level
of improvement seen at two months. Virtually identical findings have been reported for other sulphonylureas.

The Frenchman Auguste Loubatieres devoted much of his
life to the development of sulphonylureas and he had previously reported that if insulin and a sulphonylurea were given
to animals the hypoglycaemic effect was greater than when
insulin was given alone, i.e. the sulphonylurea potentiated the
action of insulin.

Combining these two sets of observations it has been
concluded that sulphonylureas have an action which is in
addition to their ability to promote insulin secretion. This has
been termed an extra-pancreatic mechanism of action.

The nature of this extra-pancreatic mechanism of action is
uncertain but recent work suggests that sulphonylurea administration can lead to an increase in the number of insulin receptors on cells. Thus, there are more sites for insulin action and
we might explain the findings above by postulating that
although in the six month oral glucose tolerance test insulin
was present in the same amount it was able to act more
efficiently due to an increase in insulin receptors.

Workers in the field fall into two camps—those who

attribute long term sulphonylurea effects to an extra-pancreatic effect, and a second group who deny or are doubtful about the existence of this effect. Naturally the effect cannot be denied unless an alternative explanation of the finding is presented. The doubters, and the term is used scientifically rather than derogatorily, would argue that at base-line, insulin secretion is inappropriately low for the blood glucose concentration and at 6 months, when the same insulin secretion is found for a lower blood glucose concentration, then this actually constitutes an improvement in secretion. The corollary of this argument is that sulphonylureas work by increasing the sensitivity of the B cell to factors, particularly glucose, which cause insulin secretion.

Which patients are suitable for sulphonylurea therapy?

Which diabetic patients are suitable for sulphonylurea therapy? We have already drawn attention to one basic feature of these patients which is that they must be able to secrete some insulin. In other words they must not be insulin-dependent. Earlier in this chapter we dealt with the role of diet in treating non-insulin-dependent diabetes. Sulphonylureas are used in patients who do not achieve satisfactory blood glucose concentrations on diet. This may take the form of a complete non-response to diet from the outset–in jargon, 'primary dietary failures', or when a period of satisfactory control of blood glucose is followed by a deterioration— 'secondary dietary failures'. In patients who are under their ideal body weight or near normal body weight this is a logical step, but in obese subjects, many of whom do not achieve a satisfactory response to diet, the use of sulphonylureas is more problematical. For reasons which are not clearly understood sulphonylureas may lead to an increase in weight in patients to whom they are given. Since this is the very thing one wants to avoid in these patients the use of sulphonylureas is debat-able. Faced with a situation, however, where an obese patient is being treated with a diet, but not well-controlled, a judge-ment has to be made as to which is the most harmful, obesity or persistent hyperglycaemia. At this point many physicians would opt to introduce a drug into the treatment.

There are other occasions when sulphonylureas are used to

treat patients although the rationale of their use is less clear-cut. At times a sulphonylurea may be given to a newly diagnosed non-insulin-dependent diabetic patient. This would seem to go against the principle that all such patients should have a period of treatment with a diet. Usually they are used at diagnosis in a group of patients who are presumed to be primary dietary failures. The grounds for this assumption are empirical. The history of diabetes may be short, the severity of symptoms marked, or weight loss and ketonuria may be present. None of these grounds are secure and the decision arises from the experience of the prescribing physician. The dangers of this approach are that experience may be governed by recent memory. Remembering that the last three patients who presented like this failed to respond to diet may influence the physician to skip the important dietary stage of treatment.

Sulphonylureas may control diabetes for a variable period of time but when control fails a decision on further treatment with insulin is necessary. This decision may be delayed because of social circumstances, age, or other associated diseases, and it should be pointed out that symptoms are not always a major complaint in these people. In most clinics, therefore, there is a small group of patients in whom diabetic control is poor, despite sulphonylurea therapy, but who do not have marked symptoms of uncontrolled diabetes.

Which sulphonylurea?

Choosing a sulphonylurea for an individual patient is a decision which the pharmaceutical industry spend large sums of money in an attempt to influence. Most clinics adopt the policy that it is better to gain experience with two or three sulphonylureas rather than try the lot. Within the sulphonylureas, however, there are some important differences between drugs. Tolbutamide and chlorpropamide were the first drugs to gain widespread clinical use and are often referred to as 'first generation sulphonylureas'. All the remainder of the sulphonylureas were introduced at a later date, for this reason they are termed 'second generation sulphonylureas'. The advantage of second generation drugs, if it is an advantage, is that they are more potent. A smaller amount of the drug is needed to produce the same effect as a large dose of a first generation drug. It should be stated that both tolbutamide and chlorpropamide have stood the test of time well and still have a large share of the oral hypoglycaemic agent market.

The second and more important difference between sulphonylureas is the division into short-acting and long-acting. Tolbutamide and glipizide are short-acting drugs while the remainder are long-acting. The significance of this distinction is that accumulation of a long-acting drug is more probable and this has implications for their use in the elderly. This point will be taken up again later.

Side-effects

Side-effects of sulphonylureas include a skin rash following instigation of therapy. This is a typical drug eruption, widespread over the body and consisting of small raised red spots or more widespread erythema. If it occurs there is little point in trying another sulphonylurea since they cross-react. The drug should be stopped immediately when the rash will begin to fade. So far we have considered all the drugs in this group as sulphonylureas but in strict chemical terms acetohexamide and glymidine are not sulphonylureas. For this reason they may not cause a skin rash in those patients allergic to other members of the group and therefore they should be tried in such patients.

The most important, since it is the most dangerous, side-effect is hypoglycaemia. Two factors influence the occurrence of hypoglycaemia. As with patients on insulin, loss of appetite with subsequent decreased food intake makes hypoglycaemia more likely. Secondly, anything which impairs breakdown and excretion of the drug leading to accumulation makes hypoglycaemia a possibility. Sulphonylureas are metabolised and excreted by the liver and kidneys. Prescribing any drug in liver disease is a highly specialised subject and will not be considered further. Of greater importance is a deterioration in renal function. Two groups especially at risk are those patients with diabetic small vessel disease which affects the kidney, and the elderly since renal function declines with age. Prevention of hypoglycaemia depends upon an awareness of these 'at risk' groups. In general terms, it is safer for the elderly to take a short-acting sulphonylurea. This is less of a problem when diagnosis occurs in the elderly since they are likely to be started on tolbutamide. It is more of a problem when the patient started chlorpropamide or glibenclamide at the age of 55 and still takes it at the age of 70. They may have lost touch with the diabetic clinic or be given the enthusiastic advice to 'carry-on' when they attend the clinic. Whatever the reason the nurse visiting the patient should be aware of the dangers.

Sulphonylurea-induced hypoglycaemia is rare but may be devastating. It is not to be viewed in the same light as insulin-induced hypoglycaemia and should not be treated at home or in a Casualty Department by a single injection of intravenous glucose or a few dextrasols. Patients who develop hypoglycaemia during sulphonylurea therapy need observation for a minimum of 24 hours. We said earlier that the possible mechanism of action of sulphonylureas was to enhance the secretion of insulin and to increase the sensitivity of the B cell to glucose. To treat this type of hypoglycaemia with intravenous glucose may further stimulate insulin secretion. Glucagon injection is not an alternative since glucagon also stimulates insulin secretion. The correct treatment is an intravenous infusion and and careful monitoring, and this may be necessary for 48 hours. Even with this treatment, success is not guaranteed as the infusion may cause insulin to pour out of the B cell with risk of hypoglycaemia as soon as the infusion is discontinued. The principle of this treatment is to maintain the blood glucose concentration while the effect of the drug wears off. An alternative which may sometimes be necessary is administration of diazoxide which blocks insulin release. The important lesson is that treatment of sulphonylurea-induced hypoglycaemia necessitates hospital admission.

There is a second point concerning sulphonylurea-induced hypoglycaemia to which attention should be drawn. The brain is entirely dependent upon a constant supply of glucose for metabolism. If the supply is decreased as during hypoglycaemia, neurological changes may be the major presenting signs. This is again particularly true in the elderly when pre-existing arterial disease may make certain areas of the brain more sensitive to hypoglycaemia. Thus, the major presenting sign of hypoglycaemia may be an apparent stroke and it is therefore important in such patients to measure the blood glucose concentration. Treatment of the hypoglycaemia usually restores normal cerebral function and this should not be missed. Of course, there are elderly patients who do have a cerebrovascular accident as the primary event when hypoglycaemia may ensue as a result of a decreased intake. In these patients the signs of the stroke will not resolve on treatment of the hypoglycaemia. Nevertheless damaged cerebral tissue may be further harmed by decreasing its nutrient supply and the hypoglycaemia should be treated promptly. Reservations have already been expressed above about treatment of sulphonylurea-induced hypoglycaemia by glucose ingestion or injection. This should not be taken to mean that nothing should be done beyond calling an ambulance. Glucose administration should be undertaken if only to buy a little time for the journey to hospital.

Some patients taking chlorpropamide develop facial flushing after drinking alcohol. It is an interesting side-effect of the drug but while it is interesting to the doctor it can be embarrassing to the patient. If troublesome an alternative sulphonylurea may be used. Diabetic patients are often uncertain of whether they should drink alcohol, and if they do, whether they should admit as much to the doctor. They often have to be asked directly whether they develop facial flushing with alcohol ingestion.

A more important side-effect of chlorpropamide is in preventing water excretion. This does not occur commonly but it is important that it is detected. Oedema is not a feature but the water is held in the circulation thus diluting serum electrolytes. A rather non-specific clinical syndrome emerges with weakness, lassitude, and it may progress to confusion and coma. A simple measurement of the serum sodium usually provides the answer. The normal range for serum sodium is 134–146 mmol/l but in this chlorporpamide-induced inappropriate anti-diuretic hormone syndrome, serum sodium is low and sometimes may decline to less than 110 mmol/l. Interestingly, this side-effect is not shared by some of the other sulphonylureas and indeed glibenclamide may have a mild diuretic action.

A discussion of the side-effects of sulphonylureas should not detract from their usefulness in treating non-insulin-dependent diabetes. Side-effects are uncommon, nevertheless awareness of their existence is a major part of early detection or better still, prevention.

Biguanides

The hypoglycaemic action of Guanidine was noted about 1920. However, there appeared to be considerable liver toxicity with early diguanide derivatives. The early part of this century was not a good time to introduce hypoglycaemic agents. Insulin had just been used for the first time and it must have seemed that a cure for diabetes had been found. Simple replacement therapy should do the trick and, indeed, it clearly did in the patients who would have previously died in ketoacidosis. Much later, it would become apparent that the mortality from ketoacidosis was being replaced by morbidity and mortality from diabetic complications. With the dawning of this realisation and the implied corollary that simple insulin replacement therapy was not to be a complete answer, interest in oral hypoglycaemic agents was reawakened.

Shortly after the introduction of the sulphonylureas came the biguanides—phenformin, metformin and buformin. It was readily apparent from the outset that, as for the sulphonylureas, they did not work in patients with no insulin secretion. In contrast to sulphonylureas, however, the hypoglycaemic effect of biguanides was not produced through stimulation of insulin secretion. The possibilities this raised were important. Firstly, they could be tried in patients who did not respond to sulphonylureas since this would not predict whether a patient would respond to biguanides, and secondly, there were now two groups of oral agents working in different ways and this allowed them to be used in combination, where one type alone might be only partially successful in controlling diabetes.

How do they work?

An early reported side-effect of biguanide administration was anorexia, sometimes accompanied by nausea and vomiting. Following this observation it was suggested that they may have an effect upon absorption from the gastrointestinal tract. Later work showed that glucose absorption was impaired, also absorption of amino acids, other sugars, and some vitamins. Here was part of the mechanism by which a hypoglycaemic effect was produced.

Biguanides were also of major interest to the physiologists

and biochemists. In a large number of animal experiments they were shown to cause a decrease in production of glucose by the liver. This inhibition of hepatic gluconeogenesis would again explain in part a hypoglycaemic action, and recent confirmation in humans of this effect has been obtained.

A third effect was noted by Sir John Butterfield and his colleagues. They found that biguanides increased the utilisation of glucose by the human forearm. In other words, biguanides increased the entry of glucose into cells of the tissues hence lowering blood glucose concentration. This effect is perhaps the most controversial of the three and varying results have been obtained with some groups reporting no effect upon peripheral utilisation of glucose. Nevertheless, the three mechanisms contribute to a hypoglycaemic effect although it should not be thought that each contributes one-third to the effect.

A question which has puzzled workers in the field is how can a single drug produce such diverse effects. The answer has been a long time in coming but it appears that biguanides bind to membranes of cells and block metabolic processes. In other words they are rather non-specific drugs, and, fortuitously, a major result is the lowering of blood glucose. It is a version of somebody's law that for 20 years biguanides were used clinically without a clear idea of the underlying mechanism of action, and just as we begin to understand the latter the clinical uses decline. The reasons for this will be discussed later.

Which biguanide?

This is a question which does not arise in some countries. Of the three biguanides only phenformin used to be available for routine clinical use in the U.S.A. This is no longer so since it was officially withdrawn in the late 1970s. Metformin and buformin were never introduced in the U.S.A. so currently no biguanide is available. In Europe, a number of countries also withdrew phenformin but in the majority of these countries metformin and buformin remain available. In the U.K. buformin has never been extensively used, phenformin was used widely for many years but currently availability is limited, and only metformin is in widespread clinical use.

It is impossible to consider the question 'Which biguanide?' without considering the side-effects of the drug. This is done below, and it emerges that metformin is safest and as effective as either of the other two. Phenformin and buformin should be reserved for patients in whom metformin produces intolerable side-effects.

Which patients are suitable for biguanide therapy?

If we think back to Chapter 1 and the aetiology of non-insulin-dependent diabetes in obese subjects, we recall that obese diabetics, if given oral glucose, have an insulin response greater than normal weight, normal subjects—they are hyper-insulinaemic. Experimental evidence suggests that high circulating insulin concentrations may have a causative role in producing arterial disease. Thus in these subjects the aim of treatment should be to reduce blood glucose and also to reduce serum insulin. In earlier discussion of the sulphonylureas, attention was drawn to the finding that sulphonylureas reduce blood glucose but leave insulin unchanged and at times may even increase insulin secretion. Clearly their use is not entirely appropriate in obese patients.

Equally clearly the best means of lowering glucose and insulin is by diet and few if any obese subjects should be given oral agents before an adequate trial of diet. There remains, however, a group of obese diabetics who are non-insulin-dependent, in whom diet, for whatever reason, fails to lower blood glucose. Faced with this recurring problem the biguanides, which lower blood glucose without stimulating insulin secretion, are a valuable adjunct to therapy. Indeed, by lowering blood glucose the stimulus to insulin secretion is reduced and circulating insulin is lowered.

There is an additional, slightly sadistic, indication for biguanides in obese subjects. The side-effects of anorexia and nausea may improve the adherence to a weight-reducing diet. A biguanide combined with a weight-reducing diet may successfully control diabetes when dietary therapy alone has failed.

The second major group of patients who are given biguanides are those in whom diabetic control is inadequate on sulphonylureas. In this group of patients the combination of drugs acting in different ways may result in good control of diabetes. It should be clearly stated that this is what is meant by combination therapy and there is never any point in giving a patient two sulphonylureas, or two biguanides.

Side-effects

Anorexia, nausea and vomiting have been discussed. Other side-effects originating in the gastrointestinal system are a metallic taste in the mouth and diarrhoea. During metformin therapy diarrhoea can be troublesome and many patients must have undergone sigmoidoscopy and barium enema to investigate the symptom because of failure to realise that it was caused by metformin. Incapacity due to metformin-induced diarrhoea is probably one of the few reasons for prescribing phenformin or buformin. Two important side-effects of biguanides deserve further consideration—the development of lactic acidosis during biguanide therapy, and the results of the UGDP study.

Soon after phenformin was introduced attention was drawn to the occurrence of a metabolic acidosis not due to ketoacidosis, occurring during phenformin therapy. To date there are over 300 reports of lactic acidosis associated with biguanide therapy in the literature of which the vast majority are associated with phenformin therapy. This is a serious condition with a mortality around 50 per cent. All patients taking phenformin have abnormally elevated lactate concentrations in the blood and so must be considered potential candidates for developing lactic acidosis. It would seem that a further insult can tip the patient into acidosis. This further insult may take an acute form such as the development of a myocardial infarction or a severe infection, or alternatively may have a more chronic onset. The latter is likely to occur if metabolism and/or excretion of the drug is impaired. Accumulation of the drug then leads to the risk of lactic acidosis developing. This accumulation is particularly likely to occur in the elderly and those with diabetic kidney complications. Lactic acidosis is more likely to occur in patients in whom co-existing disease is present which also tends to increase blood lactate concentrations; such diseases include chronic respiratory disease, and cardiovascular disease.

Of the cases reported in the literature few have been

associated with metformin and, in the majority of these cases, metformin administration was totally inappropriate, being given to anuric patients. This discrepancy between the two biguanides is not due to disporportionate risks of prescribing. Thus, in terms of this side-effect metformin is to be preferred to phenformin. Buformin occupies an intermediate position.

At the conclusion of this section it is appropriate to return to the American study known as the University Group Diabetes Program (UGDP), since the findings of this study applied to both a sulphonylurea—tolbutamide, and a biguanide—phenformin.

Ten reputable centres in the United States took part in the study and the non-insulin-dependent diabetic patients were allocated to different treatments. About 200 patients were in each group treated by placebo, a fixed dose of insulin, a variable dose of insulin, tolbutamide, or phenformin. The findings with regard to the oral agents was sufficiently alarming to warrant early publication and withdrawal of the drugs. There was a significant increase in mortality in both these groups compared with the placebo-taking group and this was most marked for deaths from cardiovascular causes.

Since publication of the findings debate has raged with analysis and re-analysis of results, argument and counterargument. The major criticism of the study from European Diabetologists has concerned, not the mortality in the treated groups, but the low mortality in the placebo group. Thus, it has been suggested that the mortality in the treated groups was not higher than would be expected but that the mortality in the placebo group was lower that that encountered in other studies of diabetic patients. An eminent group of statisticians addressed this point and indicated certain problems with regard to the initial allocation of patients to groups but did not feel that the results were invalid because of this.

There seems no way to resolve these arguments without a repetition of the study and currently there is a multi-centre study in the U.K. addressing the problem. In general terms, European Diabetologists have largely ignored the study findings at least with regard to their prescribing habits. In the U.S.A. acceptance of the findings has been more widespread and a number of reputable centres do not use oral hypoglycaemic agents because of the outcome of the UGDP study.

THEORETICAL ASPECTS OF INSULIN THERAPY

It is important that the aims of therapy are clearly stated. A primary aim is relief of dis-ease, or an improvement in well being through relief of symptoms. The majority of symptoms arise from the increased blood glucose concentration which exceeds the renal threshold. Polyuria, followed by thirst, plus or minus dehydration ensues. Recognition of thirst by a patient does not always follow a close relationship with a rise in blood glucose. This is clear from the patients who complain only of pruritis vulvae or balanitis and may deny thirst altogether or only recall it if asked specifically about the symptom. Factors which lower blood glucose will usually alleviate symptoms and insulin is highly successful in this respect.

There is an additional aim to therapy, however, in attempting to prevent disabling complications of long term diabetes. The evidence that good control of blood glucose is important in this respect is reviewed in the next section and the reader can assess how strong the case is. Most people involved in the treatment of diabetes accept that some degree of blood glucose control is important or to put this another way, no-one would deliberately assign a patient to poor control. How rigorous should be our attempts to control blood glucose is debatable, with some doctors advocating tight control and others being less rigorous.

Good control of blood glucose by diet or by oral agents is entirely feasible and a logical aim of therapy. With insulin therapy, however, this good control of blood glucose is not always attainable without the risk of hypoglycaemia and it is this latter factor which causes some physicians concern. What is good control? Obtaining and maintaining blood glucose concentrations which are normal or as near normal as possible without frequent recurrent hypoglycaemic attacks. The range for blood glucose concentrations throughout the day in normal subjects is from 3.5 mmol/l to 8 mmol/l depending upon meals. In keeping blood glucose concentration within this range, normal people have two distinct advantages. Firstly, insulin is secreted from the B cell of the islets of Langerhans in the pancreas promptly following meals. In this respect the rise in blood glucose concentration after food is important but is not the only factor responsible. Amino acids absorbed from the gut also stimulate insulin secretion and there are also hormonal factors released by the gut which on arrival at the pancreas enhance insulin secretion. Following absorption of food, the rise in blood glucose concentration peaks and then begins to fall. At this time the fall in blood glucose reduces the stimulation to insulin secretion and this begins to diminish. Thus insulin secretion is finely linked to changes in blood glucose concentration (Fig. 2.7). The second advantage which normal subjects possess is that the insulin is secreted into the portal system and passes directly to the liver. We have already learnt from the biochemistry (Ch. 1) that the liver has many important metabolic functions, thus high concentrations of insulin arrive at exactly the site where they are most needed. A proportion of the insulin which reaches the liver (about 50 per cent) is broken down in the liver and the remaining 50 per cent passes through the liver and on to other tissues. Thus, there is a gradient in insulin concentration between the liver and other tissues.

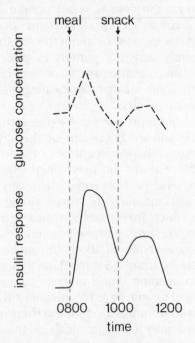

Figure 2.7 The insulin response to changes in blood glucose concentration following a meal and snack in a non-diabetic subject

The first of these mechanisms is very important when we consider insulin-dependent diabetic people. When insulin is given via bolus injection into subcutaneous tissues there is no means by which release from tissues is dependent or linked to the prevailing blood glucose concentration. The absorption of insulin is governed mainly by the physical form of the administered insulin and to a lesser extent by the site of injection and the bloodflow around the injection site. Since insulin release from the injection site is not linked to blood glucose concentration the level of circulating insulin after meals may be low or during hypoglycaemia may be high, situations which do not occur in normal people. The aims of insulin therapy must be, therefore, to choose insulins and times of injection, and frequency of injections which will deliver insulin into the circulation in amounts which are appropriate to the blood glucose concentration. In other words the rate of insulin delivery must be pre-planned in our choice of insulin regimens.

One of the best ways we can approach this is to examine the response of insulin secretion in normal subjects during a day (Fig. 2.8). The picture we see is of a continual low secretion of insulin with rapid rises with meals. Insulin secretion is also rapidly reduced when blood glucose falls after meals. Since

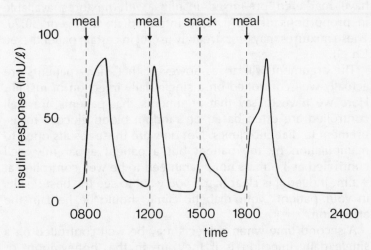

Figure 2.8 Circulating insulin levels over a 24 hour period in a normal person. Note that there is always a small amount present but this rises rapidly after food.

the aim of therapy is to obtain normal blood glucose concentrations, mimicking this pattern would clearly be a logical approach. We must next consider the tools available to achieve this.

There are many insulin preparations on the market but broadly they fall into three main groups termed rapid acting, intermediate acting and long acting (Tables 5.3–5.5).

In theory, the best imitation of the normal pattern could be achieved by giving a long-acting insulin to mimic the continual low secretion of insulin and injections of rapid-acting insulin to imitate the responses with meals, and some groups of workers have achieved notable success using Ultratard as the long-acting insulin and Actrapid three times a day. Anyone who has tried to persuade a patient from one injection a day to two injections per day will appreciate the difficulties of further persuading the patient to inject three times per day. In view of these difficulties a compromise may be accepted. Breakfast and the evening meal may be dealt with by injections of rapid-acting insulin while the midday meal and the bed-time snack through to breakfast are covered by two injections of intermediate-acting insulin. Thus the patient receives two injections per day of a mixture of rapid and intermediate-acting insulin. To facilitate this a number of pharmaceutical companies have marketed pre-mixed insulins with mixtures available in proportions of 50:50 rapid:intermediate acting or 30:70. These mixtures may be extremely useful in certain patients (see Ch. 5).

The argument will arise, however, that many patients are actually well controlled on a single daily injection of insulin. Here we have to say that arguments that patients are well controlled are often based on random blood glucose measurement in diabetic clinics. Not only are these results open to manipulation by the patient but a patient apparently well controlled at 3 p.m. is not guaranteed to be well controlled at 9 a.m. Indeed it is clear that if you want to see the best results in your patients your diabetic clinic should be held in the afternoon.

A second time when subjects may be well controlled on a single daily injection is if they are in the 'honeymoon' or remission period of diabetes as often occurs in children. Following diagnosis of diabetes and commencement of insulin the aim of therapy is to obtain normal blood glucose concentrations, mimicking this pattern would clearly be a logical approach. We must next consider the tools available to achieve this.

There are many insulin preparations on the market but broadly they fall into three main groups termed rapid acting, intermediate acting and long acting (Tables 5.3–5.5).

In theory, the best imitation of the normal pattern could be achieved by giving a long-acting insulin to mimic the continual low secretion of insulin and injections of rapid-acting insulin to imitate the responses with meals, and some groups of workers have achieved notable success using Ultratard as the long-acting insulin and Actrapid three times a day. Anyone who has tried to persuade a patient from one injection a day to two injections per day will appreciate the difficulties of further persuading the patient to inject three times per day. In view of these difficulties a compromise may be accepted. Breakfast and the evening meal may be dealt with by injections of rapid-acting insulin while the midday meal and the bed-time snack through to breakfast are covered by two injections of intermediate-acting insulin. Thus the patient receives two injections per day of a mixture of rapid and intermediate-acting insulin. To facilitate this a number of pharmaceutical companies have marketed pre-mixed insulins with mixtures available in proportions of 50:50 rapid:intermediate acting or 30:70. These mixtures may be extremely useful in certain patients (see Ch. 5).

The argument will arise, however, that many patients are actually well controlled on a single daily injection of insulin. Here we have to say that arguments that patients are well controlled are often based on random blood glucose measurement in diabetic clinics. Not only are these results open to manipulation by the patient but a patient apparently well controlled at 3 p.m. is not guaranteed to be well controlled at 9 a.m. Indeed it is clear that if you want to see the best results in your patients your diabetic clinic should be held in the afternoon.

A second time when subjects may be well controlled on a single daily injection is if they are in the 'honeymoon' or remission period of diabetes as often occurs in children. Following diagnosis of diabetes and commencement of insulin

The first of these mechanisms is very important when we consider insulin-dependent diabetic people. When insulin is given via bolus injection into subcutaneous tissues there is no means by which release from tissues is dependent or linked to the prevailing blood glucose concentration. The absorption of insulin is governed mainly by the physical form of the administered insulin and to a lesser extent by the site of injection and the bloodflow around the injection site. Since insulin release from the injection site is not linked to blood glucose concentration the level of circulating insulin after meals may be low or during hypoglycaemia may be high, situations which do not occur in normal people. The aims of insulin therapy must be, therefore, to choose insulins and times of injection, and frequency of injections which will deliver insulin into the circulation in amounts which are appropriate to the blood glucose concentration. In other words the rate of insulin delivery must be pre-planned in our choice of insulin regimens.

One of the best ways we can approach this is to examine the response of insulin secretion in normal subjects during a day (Fig. 2.8). The picture we see is of a continual low secretion of insulin with rapid rises with meals. Insulin secretion is also rapidly reduced when blood glucose falls after meals. Since

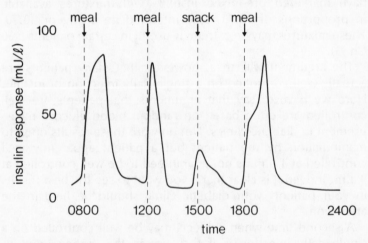

Figure 2.8 Circulating insulin levels over a 24 hour period in a normal person. Note that there is always a small amount present but this rises rapidly after food.

therapy over the next few months there may occur a decrease in insulin requirement. A new level of requirement is arrived at and may last for months or even years. If we examine the record of these patients we see during this time that blood glucose control is excellent and urine tests are regularly negative for glycosuria. This is the honeymoon period of diabetes and is characterised by some recovery of insulin secretion. At times this may be to a degree where insulin can be discontinued for a short time but more often it means that we need only get the administered dose approximately right and the patient's own secretion will make up to the correct dose and keep blood glucose control excellent.

To be fair to the once-a-day injection protagonists we should say that the evidence that twice-a-day insulin obtains any better control than once-a-day insulin is slight, and although we would recommend more than one injection per day in young and middle-aged adults, this may not be feasible in the elderly or very young.

It is obvious that when insulin therapy is pre-planned as it must always be, a certain rigidity of meals creeps in. During twice daily injections, two of the main meals are covered by rapid-acting insulin given immediately prior to meals and this allows a certain latitude in timing. The midday meal, however, is governed by insulin injected several hours previously and the regimen is arranged to provide insulin amounts appropriate to the eating of a meal. In view of this there is considerably less latitude in the timing of this meal. With once a day insulin the evening meal must also be added to this reservation. If blood glucose is to be kept down after the evening meal, the concentration of insulin will be high at this time. Failure to eat the meal on time is likely to result in hypoglycaemia. That this does not occur more commonly can be attributed to the fact that the patient is not particularly well controlled at this time.

Hypoglycaemia is the single most common side-effect of insulin therapy and is of such importance that a section is devoted to it in Chapter 6. Other side-effects occurring during insulin therapy are considered in Chapter 5. For the remainder of this section we want to consider one further point—the dose of insulin.

The dose of insulin per day which an insulin-dependent

diabetic patient needs is determined empirically. By this is meant that the dose is increased until blood glucose is well controlled. It is important when starting a patient on insulin that we begin with a small dose of 16–24 u/day. This will avoid severe hypoglycaemia in a few patients who are insulin-sensitive. If this dose fails to control blood glucose the dose is increased daily until control is achieved. Prediction of the dose is almost impossible but the daily dose needed rarely exceeds 1 u/kg. In a recent study in our clinic, the average daily dose of insulin in 50 adult diabetic patients was 50 units per day. At the Birmingham Children's Hospital the average daily dose of 35 children aged 5–17 was 55 units per day. Not too much should be made of this figure since we do not know if the degree of control was the same in the children and the adults, but they highlight one important point. The amount of insulin produced by the human pancreas each day is equivalent to approximately 28 units. Why is it that replacement therapy for insulin deficiency requires on average twice this figure and sometimes considerably more? Discussion of this point is outside the scope of this text but one aspect of it should be considered further.

The main insulins used in the treatment of diabetes are pig insulin or beef insulin. Recently human insulin has been made available either by chemical modification of pig insulin (semi-synthetic) or by bacterial synthesis (biosynthetic). Pig insulin differs from human insulin in only one amino acid while beef insulin differs by three amino acids. Before the advent of highly purified insulins all patients treated by insulin developed antibodies to the proteins which came from different species. Considerable research has gone into elucidating the significance of antibodies to insulin and they seem to have remarkably little effect. Since they bind injected insulin the presence of antibodies in a patient may result in short-acting insulin being converted into long-acting insulin in the blood. The antibodies will slowly release insulin. Since some of the bound insulin may be destroyed it should be expected that patients with lots of antibodies would need more administered insulin. This is by no means certain; however some studies support this view and the presence of antibodies may therefore affect the dose of insulin needed. Interestingly, the early studies with human insulin also produced antibodies and this

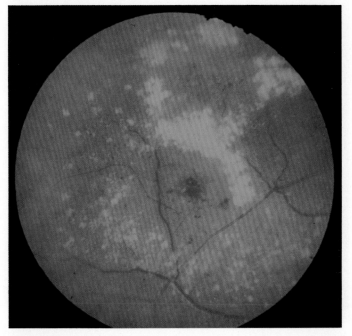

Colour Plate 1:
Background retinopathy: The predominant feature is the hard
exudates but in the centre, microaneurysms (small red dots) and
haemorrhage can be seen.

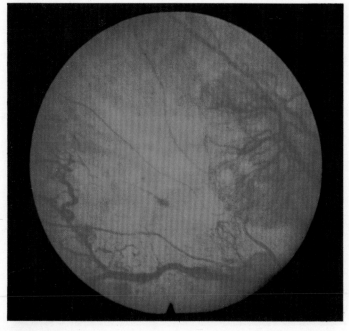

Colour Plate 2:
Proliferative retinopathy: Extensive new vessel growth shown right as arcades of fragile, thin vessels. Further examples of abnormal vessels are shown bottom, left.

may have been related to the method of altering the time course of action rather than the insulin itself.

Summary

The aims of insulin therapy are to relieve symptoms and prevent the development of diabetic complications. Currently most physicians would aim for good blood glucose control as a means of achieving both these aims. The logical approach is to attempt to mimic circulating insulin patterns in non-diabetic people. Twice or three times daily injections of insulin may do this best although in some patients, e.g. the elderly or very young children, once daily injections may have to be used.

DOES DIABETIC CONTROL MATTER

The question under consideration in this section is really whether good control of diabetes can reduce the incidence of the disabling complications and decrease the mortality attributable to diabetes. What is not in doubt is that relief of acute symptoms of diabetes, thirst, polyuria, weight loss etc. is well worthwhile. All treating diabetes would consider it important to relieve pruritis vulvae or balanitis. In the long run, however, does the degree of control of diabetes influence whether the diabetic patient develops retinopathy, neuropathy, arterial disease, or renal failure?

The answer to this question is fundamental to the approach of all concerned in the management of patients with diabetes. It is readily apparent that acute symptoms can be relieved without necessarily obtaining good glucose control. If the treatment does not influence the development of complications, then perhaps the only aim of therapy should be symptomatic relief. If, on the other hand, diabetic patients who are well controlled develop less in the way of complications then all our efforts should go into improving the standard of control. In view of the central nature of this question it is surprising that no clear answer has emerged. In this section the evidence that good control is important will be reviewed.

Let us look first of all at the evidence from experiments with animals. Animals such as mice or rats can readily be made diabetic by giving injections of the chemical alloxan or strep-tozotocin. These chemicals destroy the B cells of the islets of Langerhans and thus make the animal insulin deficient. The animals can then be given daily injections of insulin and development of complications and the effects of treatment studied. Thus has been created an 'animal model' for insulin-dependent diabetes. With animals, however, treatment can be taken one stage further than with humans and two groups can be studied, in one of which diabetes is controlled well and in the other poor control is allowed. Most of the evidence from animal experiments suggests that the well-controlled animals develop less in the way of complications than poorly controlled animals. Indeed if the animals are returned to a normal state by giving them back insulin-producing cells (transplanting islets from a sister animal), any complications which have developed can be seen to regress.

On the face of it the case already seems proven—good control does prevent complications developing. It is not quite that straightforward. Firstly, it really is not clear whether the complications which animals develop are identical to those which develop in humans. Secondly, the animals were made diabetic by a chemical, therefore the diabetes cannot be subject to any genetic influences. If these influences play a part in human diabetes then the animal model created cannot be considered a good model for human diabetes.

In view of this lingering doubt over animal experiments what can be deduced from studies in human diabetics? Many studies have been performed attempting to relate control and complications. A majority have entailed studying patients with lesser and more marked degrees of diabetic complications, by thumbing back through the medical records and looking up blood or urine tests on attendance at clinic. Many of the studies are not worth the paper they were written on and the American physician Dr Harvey Knowles did the diabetic world a great service in 1964 by collating over 300 such studies, thus saving us all considerable time which might otherwise have been spent examining each study in detail. Most of the studies, (over 200) did not contain sufficient data for analysis. Of the studies which Dr Knowles considered worthy of analysis, 50 studies supported a relationship between control and complications, in 25 a relationship did not appear to exist, and in 10 the case was non-proven. One major study since that time deserves further consideration since it has attracted much publicity. The distinguished Belgian diabetologist, Dr Jean Pirart, reported the results of 4400 patients attending his clinic between 1947 and 1973. Through the years, patients were assessed for the development of diabetic complications and the degree of blood glucose control was recorded. The clear picture which emerged (and there is much more of interest in the report) was that patients with good control of blood glucose developed less diabetic complications. Case proved?—alas no!! Other explanations can be put forward to explain the results. Let us put forward an alternative explanation, not with any great conviction but rather to show that critical reading of the literature is all important. Let us assume that not all diabetics will develop complications but in any diabetic population x per cent will not and y per cent will develop severe diabetic complications. What factors can influence whether you fall into the y per cent? One, as suggested by Pirart, may be the degree of control, but it might also be something not yet identified in your genes. Now it would be possible that not only did the y per cent inherit a tendency to develop severe complications but also inherited a tendency to have difficult diabetes. If we now examine the degree of control in the two groups we would conclude erroneously that poor control *led to* severe complications, but in truth we would not be observing causation but association.

There is only one way to avoid this pitfall—when a patient starts the study they must be allocated in random manner to either a good control group or a poor control group. Not surprisingly, there are few reports along these lines. It would generally be considered unethical to deliberately control a diabetic patient poorly.

With true french flair, Dr Georges Tchobroutsky and his colleagues neatly circumvented this problem. They accepted their normal means of obtaining control—once a day insulin— as the equivalent of poor control, and put intensive effort into creating a super-good control group by twice or three times daily insulin. Once a patient had accepted to go into this study they were then randomly allocated to one of the groups. Over the two years of the study both groups showed an increase in the number of diabetic lesions in the eye but the increase was significantly greater in the group treated by once a day insulin, that is the group that had significantly worse control of blood glucose. This study is a crucial study fulfilling all the necessary requirements of random allocation of patients to two levels of diabetic control. Even this study had slight flaws, in particular some of the patients assigned to three injections per day opted for the less stringent regimen after a period in the study, and some workers have used this shifting of patients from one group to the other to reject the findings. This approach is untenable but more studies along the same lines would considerably strengthen the findings.

It is likely that many studies in the not too distant future will address this point using continuous subcutaneous insulin infusion by pumps to obtain good control of blood glucose. In one of the early studies using this technique at the Steno Hospital in Copenhagen a disturbing result was obtained. In insulin-dependent diabetic patients with evidence of complications, maintaining good diabetic control by continuous subcutaneous insulin infusion appeared to lead to a worsening of diabetic complications, particularly diabetic retinopathy. These findings cannot easily be explained but we might conclude that once long-term diabetic changes in tissues has occurred these may be irreversible and that our attempts to improve and maintain good diabetic control should be directed to the time in a patient's life when long-term damage has not occurred.

Summary

The evidence that the degree of control of blood glucose concentration affects the development of diabetic complications has been reviewed. Animal experiments support the view that poor control is associated with worse complications but lingering doubts persist regarding the similarity of complications developing in animals with those developing in man.

In humans, retrospective studies have given conflicting findings. The one prospective study supports the view that in the development of complications, diabetic control does matter. Other evidence suggests that the aim should be prevention rather than waiting until there is evidence of tissue damage before attempting to improve blood glucose control.

HOW DO WE ASSESS CONTROL OF DIABETES?

There are a number of crude indices of diabetic control. We might consider the relief from symptoms of diabetes as an improvement in control. In other situations such as during the adolescent growth spurt it is necessary to pay attention to the physical development of the patient. Poor diabetic control during adolescence may lead to a stunting of growth and this will form part of our assessment of successful diabetic treatment.

In the majority of cases, however, during the regular follow-up of diabetic patients, assessment of diabetic control will be by urine or blood glucose monitoring by the patient at home and random blood glucose estimation when they attend the diabetic clinic. Such methods of assessing control are not without their drawbacks. All are open to manipulation by the patient. Urine or blood glucose measurements by the patient at home may be manipulated either by inaccurate reading of the test or even at times by the patient maintaining a record of fictional tests. Random blood glucose measurement in the diabetic clinic may be improved by the patient through omission of the meal preceding their visit to the diabetic clinic or by a couple of days of relative starvation immediately before attending. It is well that we remember such possibilities but we must also say that the majority of our patients do wish to keep their diabetes well controlled and do approach this with honesty. We must also remember that it is exceedingly easy to blame and castigate the patient who cheats on their records. Should we not under these circumstances accept part of the blame? Such an approach to diabetes indicates a breakdown in our educational programmes. We must confess that when this situation occurs we have failed to impart to the patient the importance of good diabetic control.

In the past few years a further test of diabetic control has been introduced which is less open to manipulation by the patient. It is known that as new red blood cells are formed some of the haemoglobin which is contained within these cells combines with glucose. This fraction of the total haemoglobin is called glycosylated haemoglobin or haemoglobin A1. The amount of glycosylated haemoglobin which is formed as the red cell is born is directly proportional to the circulating glucose concentration. The life span of a red blood cell is approximately 120 days. This means that in any blood sample which we take from our patients there will be red blood cells of varying ages. Some of these will have been formed many weeks before the patient attends the diabetic clinic while some will have been formed relatively recently. The amount of glycosylated haemoglobin present in this blood sample therefore will reflect the prevailing blood glucose concentration while these cells of varying ages were formed. Thus a measurement of glycosylated haemoglobin gives some indication of the degree of blood glucose control during the preceding 6 to 8 weeks. This test is most useful as a measure of diabetic control and may reveal wide discrepancies between our clinic random blood glucose and the degree of diabetic control as measured by glycosylated haemoglobin.

The test has again confirmed how poorly controlled the majority of our insulin-dependent diabetic patients are. The upper limit of the normal range using the method of our laboratory is 8.5 per cent; most clinics have found that if glycosylated haemoglobin is measured in a group of insulin-dependent patients the average value obtained will be around 12 per cent. Some, perhaps all too few, of our patients will have levels near the upper limit of the normal range. Unfortunately some will have values of 18 to 20 per cent which indicate very poor diabetic control. The results of such a test provide a useful lever on the patient to improve control or for restabilisation of their diabetes.

It is likely that glycosylated haemoglobin measurement will be useful in resolving the debate regarding the degree of control and the development of complications. A failure of many of the studies mentioned in the previous section was that they contained no adequate long-term assessment of diabetic control. Sequential measurement of glycosylated haemoglobin will provide these data.

APPENDIX 1

Exchange List: The following amounts of foods contain 10 g carbohydrate and may be exchanged one with another to give variety to the diet.

Food	Weight	
	grams	ounces
White bread	20	$\frac{2}{3}$
Wholemeal bread	25	$\frac{3}{4}$
All Bran	20	$\frac{2}{3}$
Cornflakes	15	$\frac{1}{2}$
Weetabix	15	$\frac{1}{2}$
Plain Biscuits	15	$\frac{1}{2}$
Flour	15	$\frac{1}{2}$
Rice	30	1
Spaghetti (raw)	15	$\frac{1}{2}$
Spaghetti (tinned)	85	3
Pastry (shortcrust)	20	$\frac{2}{3}$
Milk	200	7
Yoghurt (plain)	160	$5\frac{1}{2}$
Yoghurt (fruit)	55	2
Potatoes—boiled	55	2
roast	40	$1\frac{1}{2}$
chips	30	1
crisps	25	$\frac{3}{4}$
Peas (tinned)	140	5
Baked beans	100	$3\frac{1}{2}$
Broad beans	140	5
Parsnips	75	$2\frac{1}{2}$
Apple	110	4
Banana	55	2
Grapes	70	$2\frac{1}{2}$
Pear	125	$4\frac{1}{2}$
Strawberries	160	$5\frac{1}{2}$
Drinking Chocolate	15	$\frac{1}{2}$
Lager	600 ml	1 pint
Lager—diabetic	1500 ml	$2\frac{1}{2}$ pints
Coca-cola	100 ml	$3\frac{1}{2}$ oz
Orange squash	30 ml	1 oz

3

Complications of diabetes

Introduction

Once diabetic control is achieved the fear of complications is one of the great concerns of the patient with diabetes. Diabetic complications may be acute or chronic. Acute complications are relatively rapid in onset, are usually reversible and are often due to obvious metabolic abnormalities. Hypoglycaemia and diabetic coma are examples of acute complications that are described in detail in Chapter 6. On the other hand chronic complications (Fig. 3.1) are relatively slow in onset, are mainly irreversible and their precise causes are only partly understood. Surveys have shown that in comparison with non-diabetics, patients with diabetes in western society have a two-fold increased risk of myocardial infarction, a five-fold greater amount of gangrene, a seventeen-fold higher risk of renal failure, a twenty-five fold higher risk of blindness and at least ten per cent have symptomatic disease of the peripheral nerves. Most of the chronic complications are due to structural damage to small and large blood vessels and to nerves. There is an increase of atherosclerosis causing disease of the larger arteries (macrovascular disease), a capillary lesion particularly affecting the kidneys and eyes (microvascular disease), and degeneration of peripheral and autonomic nerves (neuropathy). It should be appreciated that in any one individual

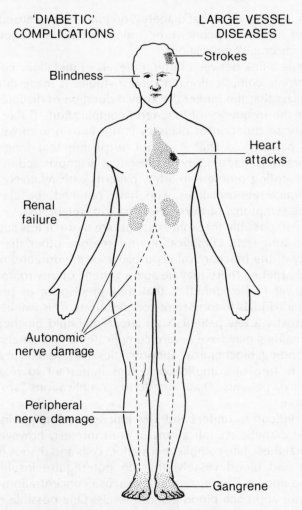

Figure 3.1 Chronic complications associated with diabetes.

patient the macrovascular and microvascular disease and the neuropathy may be occurring together so that tissue damage can arise from a combination of factors. Such a combination is important in the problems of the diabetic foot.

Direct metabolic injury

How the pathological changes of chronic complications are linked to the metabolic abnormalities of diabetes is not always known, but it is clear that diabetes, no matter how caused and whether insulin-dependent or independent, is subject to similar chronic complications.

Proving a link between different levels of metabolic control and chronic complications in clinical studies is made difficult by the fact that the longer the known duration of diabetes the greater the frequency of long-term complications (Table 3.1). The precise duration of diabetes is not known in most individual patients so that it is not surprising that long-term complications may already be present at diagnosis and may be the presenting problem in a few patients with relatively mild biochemical abnormalities who have not had the classical warning symptoms of thirst, polyuria and weight loss.

It is also possible that some patients are more or less susceptible to long-term complications for reasons other than the severity of the biochemical disturbance or the duration of the disease; that is, there may be some genetic or environmental factors yet to be identified that may predispose or protect some individuals to long-term complications. This will help to explain why a few patients with apparently mild biochemical abnormalities may have severe complications and others with longstanding biochemical abnormalities may remain free or relatively free of complications. It is important to reassure individual patients that long-term complications are not inevitable.

It is difficult to understand how glucose itself might initiate chronic diabetic complications. It is of interest, however, to note that these late complications affect cells and tissues (eyes, nerves and blood vessels) that do not require insulin for glucose uptake. The intracellular glucose concentrations may therefore approach blood glucose levels. One possible result is over-use of glucose by the cells, and in particular by the sorbitol pathway which leads to an accumulation of the sugar alcohol sorbitol within the cells. Sorbitol does not cross the cell membrane easily and is metabolised slowly. Therefore in

Table 3.1 Factors influencing development of chronic complications

Severity of metabolic disturbance
Duration of diabetes
Individual susceptibility

cells where glucose is freely permeable and where the sorbitol pathway exists there will be an accumulation of sorbitol and water within the cell. This has been best studied in the lens where swelling and coagulation of lens protein occurs with eventual cataract formation. The same sorbitol pathway is also found in peripheral nerves and in the aortic wall and may be important in causing neuropathy and even macrovascular disease. Another possible mechanism of glucose itself causing complications is by the glucose molecule itself, or a metabolite of glucose becoming attached to a protein and thereby inter-fering with its normal function or metabolism. The best example to date of such a process is glycosylation of haemo-globin which has been used to assess the degree of diabetic control. Glycosylation of haemoglobin will also to some extent interfere with oxygen transport contributing to tissue hypoxia and perhaps tissue damage. Hyperglycaemia also affects collagen, the fundamental structural protein of all connective tissue. The collagen in diabetes becomes more difficult to break down.

MICROVASCULAR DISEASE

The characteristic pathology of diabetic microvascular disease is thickening of the basement membrane in capillaries (Fig. 3.2). This membrane becomes thicker with increasing duration of diabetes, with increasing severity of diabetes and with increasing age of the individual. Thickening of the capil-lary basement membrane has been found in most tissues in diabetes and has been particularly studied in the kidney, muscle and skin. Not only is the basement membrane thicker but its biochemical structure differs from non-diabetic subjects, having a different amino acid composition and increased sugar residues attached. Raised blood glucose is associated with increased rates of synthesis of basement membrane. There is a suspicion that damage to the lining endothelial cells of the vessels may play a role in small as well as large vessel disease (see below). The loss of the pericyte cells which support the endothelial cells may be an important part of the disease process in the retina. Capillaries may become obliterated resulting in local tissue hypoxia and also abnormal

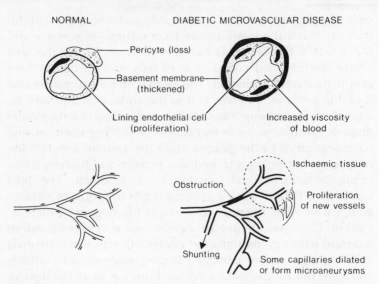

NORMAL   DIABETIC MICROVASCULAR DISEASE

Pericyte (loss)

Basement membrane (thickened)

Lining endothelial cell (proliferation)

Increased viscosity of blood

Ischaemic tissue

Obstruction

Proliferation of new vessels

Shunting

Some capillaries dilated or form microaneurysms

Figure 3.2 Characteristic pathological feature of diabetic microvascular disease.

shunting of blood directly from arterioles to venules. Such local ischaemia is likely to be the cause of many of the retinal lesions and perhaps for some of the nerve and foot lesions also. The pathology of microvascular disease should not be thought of solely in terms of structural change, but also in terms of function. The changes outlined above may be the cause of the increased leakage from capillaries in diabetes which has been shown for albumen and also for injected fluorescein in the eye. Altered permeability of the blood/nerve barrier could be important in producing nerve damage. The actual flow of blood through a capillary may also be impaired in diabetes because plasma tends to be more viscous due to increased concentrations of plasma glycoproteins, and red cells are more rigid.

LARGE VESSEL DISEASE

Atherosclerosis is not peculiar to diabetes and yet the natural history of diabetes (Ch. 1) has shown that atherosclerosis, causing problems such as myocardial infarction, stroke and gangrene, is the major cause of death. It is likely that in contrast to microvascular disease, atherosclerosis is more a feature of long-standing diabetes and is less closely related to the severity of the diabetes. Atherosclerosis appears at an earlier age, is more extensive and may develop at a more rapid rate than in non-diabetic subjects. The actual disease, however, has the same structure and is distributed among vessels in much the same way as in non-diabetic patients, with the exception of more severe peripheral arterial involvement in the legs. Both insulin-dependent and non-insulin-dependent types of diabetes are associated with increased atherosclerosis. In insulin-dependent diabetes the clinical manifestations of microvascular disease precede the development of atherosclerosis, but both processes contribute to the overall long-term complications of such patients. The effect of enhanced atherosclerosis is most obvious, however, in the non-insulin-dependent patient with most of the excess mortality due to major vessel disease affecting the heart, brain, kidneys and legs.

The impact of diabetes itself as a risk factor in cardiovascular disease is dependent upon the level of other risk factors such as genetic predisposition, obesity, hypertension and smoking. This may explain why diabetic patients in societies with low rates of atherosclerotic disease do not suffer in the same way as those in societies with higher rates. Overall diabetes is a relatively small risk factor in men, but in women the impact is much greater and eliminates most of the usual premenopausal protection from atherosclerotic disease. In women the impact of diabetes exceeds that of smoking.

Causes of atherosclerosis

Current views on the development of atherosclerosis are illustrated in Figure 3.3. Injury to the lining endothelial cells of blood vessels, however caused, leads to platelets adhering to the subendothelial structures (collagen and elastic fibres) and then large numbers of platelets aggregate together. Damaged endothelium also releases one of the clotting factors (part of the factor VIII complex). In turn platelets release many active compounds, one of which stimulates smooth muscle proliferation. The proteins that are associated with blood lipids

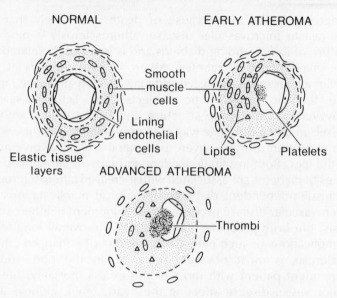

Figure 3.3 Structure of a medium-sized artery.

(especially low density lipoprotein) and insulin may act as co-factors in this proliferation. Then collagen, elastic tissue, cholesterol and lipoproteins accumulate and a patch of atheroma forms. Such patches may ulcerate and an additional blood clot forms, sometimes blocking the artery completely.

Most of these processes are enhanced in diabetes (Table 3.2) though how the initial endothelial damage occurs in diabetes is not known. Abnormalities of lipids and lipoproteins may play a role and hypertension and smoking may be additional factors in some patients. Platelet stickiness and the tendency to aggregate are increased; blood lipids may be elevated and there is a raised level of the clotting factor produced by the endothelium in diabetes. It is also true that the ability to remove the fibrin deposited in a blood clot is impaired in diabetes.

Table 3.2 Influence of diabetes on the development of atheroma

---
Increased platelet stickiness
Increased platelet aggregation
Enhanced growth of smooth muscle cells
Altered serum lipid levels
Decreased ability to remove fibrin clot

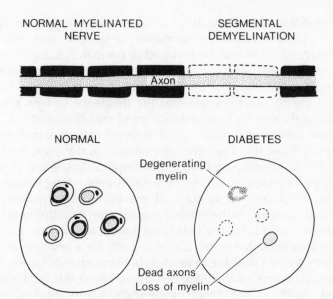

Figure 3.4 Changes in diabetic neuropathy.

NEUROPATHY

Several histological changes occur in diabetic neuropathy: loss of axons, loss of segments of the myelin sheath, proliferation of Schwann cells and increase in connective tissue elements (Fig. 3.4). The site of the primary abnormality is not known but could be within the axon, Schwann cells or the perineural space. It is likely to be a direct metabolic injury and one such mechanism may be accumulation of sorbitol which in turn may cause osmotic swelling of the cell and damage. It is also possible that there is a primary microvascular change affecting the small blood vessels supplying the nerves.

GENERAL THERAPEUTIC IMPLICATIONS

The question often asked is to what extent can control of diabetes affect the development of chronic complications? Some of the pathological changes that are thought to be of importance for vascular disease and neuropathy are reversed when diabetes is adequately controlled, for example the lipid levels, plasma viscosity, deformability of red cells and, indeed, capillary function may be restored to normal. It has also been suggested that in the early stages of long-term diabetic complications some of the structural changes, such as basement membrane thickness and the incidence of new microaneurysms, can be reversed with good metabolic control.

Both clinical observations and experimental work in diabetic animals show that the better the control of diabetes, the less the risk of developing long-term complications. Most clinical studies, however, suffer from the difficulties of long follow-up, from the failure to restore all metabolic abnormalities to normal, and from the inadequacy of the measurements of diabetic control. For the individual patient requesting reassurance that chronic complications will not be a problem in the future, it is not possible to predict, but important to stress, that if good control of diabetes can be achieved this is likely, at least, to delay the onset of clinically significant long-term complications and to minimise the problem.

Many of the established chronic complications are irreversible even though diabetic control is excellent, so that prevention and early detection of vascular disease and neuropathy are vital aspects of diabetic management. It is important to retain an optimistic approach to an individual patient with established complications because the rate of progress is very variable from patient to patient and much can be done to alleviate, arrest and minimise the damage and suffering of an individual.

SPECIFIC COMPLICATIONS OF DIABETES

The eye

Many of the structures in the eye may be affected in diabetes (Fig. 3.5). The common causes of loss of vision are cataracts and disease of the retina.

a. The lens

Cataracts, lens opacities, occur commonly in patients with diabetes and obviously contribute to the problems of visual

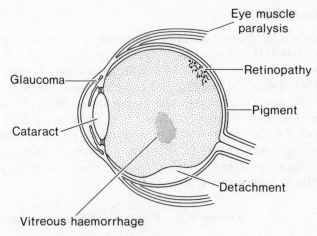

Figure 3.5 Eye problems in diabetic patients.

loss. The true, or juvenile, type of diabetic cataract is a rare, but well-documented, complication occurring early, probably at the onset of symptoms of insulin-dependent diabetes. These cataracts are invariably bilateral, with a snowflake appearance. Rapid progression with loss of vision may occur over some weeks. It is tempting to speculate that the changes in the lens, possibly glycosylation of lens protein or accumulation of sorbitol, reach such a degree in severely uncontrolled diabetes that permanent damage occurs and a cataract forms. Cataract extraction may be required at a young age. In older patients it is not entirely certain whether lens opacities are more frequent or rapid in maturation, or more severe than the non-diabetic population. There is no doubt, however, that cataract extraction is commonly required in diabetic patients and indeed the diagnosis of diabetes is often made at the eye clinic when a patient attends for consideration of cataract problems.

The management of cataract in diabetic patients is essentially the same as in the non-diabetic with the exception that artificial lenses are less frequently implanted because any co-existing or subsequently developing retinopathy cannot then be treated adequately. The results in terms of visual acuity are slightly less good than in the non-diabetic population because retinopathy may be present. Retinopathy, however, is not an absolute contraindication to surgery, as worthwhile improvement of vision may still occur after cataract surgery.

b. The retina

Microvascular disease affecting the retina is commonly found in longstanding diabetes. An increasing percentage of patients are found to have retinopathy with increasing duration of diabetes (Table 3.3), making it a common cause of blindness in middle age. Diabetic retinopathy may in fact be found when diabetes is first diagnosed (Table 3.4), suggesting that the disease has been present for a number of years before becoming symptomatic. In children, however, retinopathy is extremely rare under the age of 10 years. There are three types of diabetic retinopathy (Table 3.5).

Table 3.3 Frequency of clinical retinopathy related to known duration of diabetes

Duration of diabetes	Age of onset	Frequency of retinopathy (per cent)		
		0–29	30–59	60+
0–9 years		10	30	37
10–19 years		55	57	47
20–29 years		75	72	

Most studies of known diabetes mellitus for 30 years or more are limited to too few patients to be able to give an accurate frequency of retinopathy, but it is probably 80–90 per cent

Table 3.4 Frequency of retinopathy within a year of diagnosis of diabetes

Age (yr)	Frequency (per cent)
<40	0.6
40–59	8
60+	16
All ages	10

Table 3.5 Types of diabetic retinopathy

Type	Visual loss	Frequency in an average diabetic clinic (per cent)
Background	nil	11
Maculopathy	severe central loss	6
Proliferative retinopathy	severe	5

Background retinopathy. The majority of patients will develop a background retinopathy only. This consists of microaneurysms, dot and blot haemorrhages and hard exudates (see Colour plate 1). Hard exudates are due to fluid leaking from the dilated capillaries and from the microaneurysms, forming fatty yellowish plaques. Soft exudates or cotton wool patches are seen less frequently. These are caused by death of small areas of retina because of small vessel occlusion. The pathology of background retinopathy shows obliteration and occlusion of retinal capillaries with surrounding areas of dilated capillary shunt vessels and loss of the supporting pericytes. There is increased thickening of capillary endothelial cell basement membrane and microaneurysm formation. Intravenous fluorescein injection shows the abnormalities extremely clearly by outlining the perfused microaneurysms, by detecting sites of vascular obstruction and showing capillary leakage. Retinopathy is constantly changing and it can be shown that the average halflife of a microaneurysm is six days. The natural history of background retinopathy is very variable and early changes are potentially reversible. In most patients, mild background retinopathy advances slowly and good vision is maintained for many years. A certain number of patients will deteriorate every year, and so there is a great need for careful planned follow-up of all patients who are found to have background retinopathy.

Maculopathy. The central macular area of the retina becomes swollen due to oedema and, later, hard exudates are deposited. This type of retinopathy is most common in diabetic patients treated with an oral hypoglycaemic agent or diet alone. Severe loss of central vision results and accounts for many cases of blindness. Regular testing of visual acuity will help to detect this problem at an early stage. The peripheral retina is not usually involved and there is usually enough peripheral vision for walking. Maculopathy is not usually associated with proliferative retinopathy.

Proliferative retinopathy (Colour plate 2). This form of retinopathy differs in that the process almost invariably extends from the retina forward into the vitreous cavity, although occasional patients have proliferation on the retinal surface only. In addition to the signs of background retinopathy a network of tortuous new vessels forms on the inner surface of the retina or on the back of the vitreous. As the vitreous detaches and separates from the retina the vessels are usually pulled into the vitreous cavity. The traction on these fragile vessels leads to haemorrhage and retinal detachment. Pathologically there is proliferation of endothelial cells from the diseased retinal vessels through the inner layers of the retina into the vitreous cavity. The supporting framework of glial cells also proliferates giving a fibrous appearance.

Proliferative retinopathy occurs in all types of diabetes but particularly affects patients with longstanding insulin-dependent diabetes. The visual acuity of the patient depends upon the position of the proliferative retinopathy because if the main disease is peripheral there will be little effect, but if central, especially near the disc, visual acuity may be severely impaired. Visual acuity will also depend on the amount of vitreous haemorrhage and detachment of retina. A large vitreous haemorrhage prevents examination of the retina by ophthalmoscopy and, of course, any treatment to the retina. The natural history of severe proliferative retinopathy which has been left untreated is fairly certain progression to blindness, with 25 per cent of patients becoming blind within two years and 70 per cent within five years. A very small group of patients will have a rapidly progressive florid form; such patients are usually less than 30 years of age, have poor diabetic control and may become blind within one year. It is particularly important to recognise proliferative retinopathy before any deterioration in visual acuity has occurred. Hence the importance of examination of the eye with an ophthalmoscope, preferably through a dilated pupil. Such an examination should be done annually in those at risk—at least those with known background retinopathy or known duration of insulin-dependent diabetes for ten years or more.

Management of diabetic retinopathy

a. Medical

Good control of diabetes, adequate treatment of hypertension and avoidance of smoking may help to delay the progress of mild retinopathy, but no medical measures will be adequate to treat sight-threatening retinopathy.

b. Surgical

Photocoagulation and vitrectomy have greatly improved the outlook for patients with diabetic retinopathy, vision being maintained in about 70 per cent of patients who would otherwise have gone blind. Photocoagulation can be used to destroy (i) abnormal leaking vessels and reduce oedema of the retina, (ii) abnormal ischaemic areas of the retina which will result in regression of new vessels, and (iii) abnormal vessels directly. The two instruments used for photocoagulation are the xenon arc and the argon laser. The xenon arc produces white light which is absorbed by the pigment in the retina where it is converted into heat which destroys the adjacent retina. Xenon arc treatment produces rather large burns and so cannot be used near the centre of the eye but is useful if large areas of peripheral retina are affected. The argon laser is a green light which is absorbed by the pigment of the retina and by haemoglobin in retinal blood vessels. It can be used to burn very small areas of retina or individual lesions themselves. Sometimes three to six thousand burns are required in four or more treatments of proliferative retinopathy. Retreatment of small newly arising lesions is needed from time to time. Photocoagulation destroys retina but even when large areas of peripheral retina are treated, many patients are unaware of any loss of the field of vision. Argon laser treatment only rarely results in long-term field defects, whereas xenon arc treatment tends to leave the patient with some degree of peripheral field loss.

Vitrectomy. Attempts to remove vitreous haemorrhage and fibrous tissue in the eye and to re-attach the retina are occasionally successful in restoring some vision in advanced diabetic eye disease, provided the retina is not too severely damaged.

c. Glaucoma

Chronic simple glaucoma occurs as commonly or slightly more frequently in the diabetic compared with the general population. Its treatment is no different in the diabetic patient. Glaucoma can arise as a result of new vessels affecting the iris. The network of vessels, fibrous tissue and distorted iris, blocks the outflow of fluid from the eye. This occurs occasionally in patients who have already developed severe proliferative retinopathy. Medical treatment with acetazolamide and local steroids may be successful, but intractable pain in a blind eye can sometimes only be relieved by enucleation.

Problems in management of diabetes

Patients commonly note changes in vision at the onset of the disease and become very concerned that they may have permanent damage in the eye. Myopia, a failure of distant vision, is an initial symptom in about a third of patients and a relatively acute change in refraction may actually lead to the diagnosis of diabetes. A more disturbing symptom, however, is the failure of near vision that occurs within a few days of starting treatment with insulin. This may take some weeks to revert to normal, and in the meantime the patient may find work, or such essentials as the drawing up of insulin into a syringe, extremely difficult. It is important to make sure that the patients do not have new spectacles during such a period of stabilisation, and delay measurement of refraction for approximately two months from the start of adequate diabetic treatment.

Permanent failure of vision creates further problems in diabetic management (Table 3.6). Urine and blood glucose monitoring may be limited by a difficulty in distinguishing colours. The drawing up of insulin in a syringe requires visual acuity of 6/12 or better. Good lighting, a suitable background and a magnifying glass may be helpful. Occasionally patients are helped by a syringe with a piston limited to a predetermined dose, but the patient must be able to distinguish the difference between air and fluid in the syringe to obtain an accurate dose of insulin.

It can readily be appreciated that with increasing loss of vision the patient becomes increasingly dependent upon others in the family or community for the day to day management of diabetes. It is often an additional misfortune that the

Table 3.6 Retinopathy: effects on diabetic management

Difficulties in monitoring diabetes
Difficulties in drawing up insulin
Reduced foot care

patient with longstanding diabetes and severe visual loss will also have some loss of fine touch sensation in the finger tips so that reading in Braille is not always successful.

The kidney

Renal disease is a serious long-term complication of diabetes, particularly for the younger patient in whom it is one of the commoner causes of death. The most important pathological changes are found in the glomerulus (Fig. 3.6). Once again the basement membrane of the capillaries in the glomerulus becomes thickened. Then the glomerulus becomes increasingly replaced and destroyed by the deposition of nodules of a glycoprotein material (Kimmelsteil-Wilson nodules). The disease is aggravated in the later stages by ischaemia caused by thickening of the arteries supplying the glomerulus. There may be additional damage caused by hypertension and by renal tract infections.

Urinary tract infections may occur, because damaged renal tissue may be more susceptible, following catheterisation such as in the management of diabetic coma and because of urinary stasis when bladder emptying is faulty in autonomic neuropathy. Occasionally a severe infection of the kidney results in necrosis and sloughing of papillae, the part of the kidney substance projecting into the renal pelvis.

The first evidence of renal disease is albuminuria in the majority of patients. It is unusual to find albuminuria until after

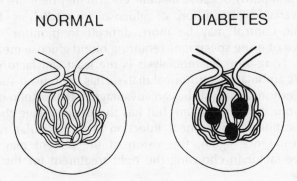

NORMAL   DIABETES

Figure 3.6 Diagram of histological changes in the diabetic glomerulus of the kidney.

15 years of diabetes and even then it may be found intermittently. Albuminuria will be present in more than half the young diabetics who have had diabetes 30 years or more. Several years may elapse, however, between the first appearance of albuminuria and any symptoms of renal impairment. Occasionally renal impairment occurs in the absence of significant albuminuria. Once renal function is impaired, progressive deterioration is inevitable although the rate is very variable from one patient to another. Fluid retention is a common symptom followed later by all the classic symptoms of uraemia. The management of the patient with terminal renal failure is made more difficult by the retinopathy which is usually present at this stage.

Management of renal disease

There is no evidence that strict metabolic control affects the progression of established renal disease but some improvement might be expected if the coexisting hypertension and renal tract infections are treated promptly and effectively. Diuretics will be needed to treat fluid retention and diet will need to be modified to a relatively low protein, high carbohydrate intake if uraemic symptoms develop.

Experience with newer methods of treatment of renal failure is limited to a few centres. Long-term dialysis is made more difficult in diabetes compared with non-diabetic patients, partly due to coexisting macrovascular disease and impaired vision and partly because diabetic control may be more erratic with variable absorption of glucose from dialysis fluids. Diabetic control may be more difficult to monitor in the absence of urine specimens requiring blood glucose measurements. Long-term haemodialysis is the least satisfactory, but chronic ambulatory peritoneal dialysis has been used successfully. Peritoneal dialysis has an advantage in that insulin can be given into the peritoneum, but has the disadvantage that the complication of peritoneal infection is a particular risk in diabetes. Once again, the vision of the patient may be a decisive factor in choosing the right treatment for the renal disease.

Renal transplantation is offered to selected patients with diabetes in some centres, but the presence of complicating

Table 3.7 Renal disease: effects on diabetic management

Increased renal threshold for glucose
Decreased insulin requirements
Aggravation of biguanide-induced lactic acidosis
Prolongation of effect of chlorpropamide
Anorexia

diseases, especially cardiovascular, and the limited resources for renal transplant programmes have seriously restricted this form of treatment. The best results have been obtained from live, related donors (Ch. 4).

Problems in the management of diabetes (Table 3.7)

Renal impairment may affect diabetic management in many ways. The renal threshold for glucose rises and so urine testing becomes a less reliable guide for blood glucose control. Drug handling may be altered—for example there is a significant prolongation of the half-life of chlorpropamide which may result in hypoglycaemia, and there is an aggravation of biguanide-induced lactic acidosis. As a consequence both chlorpropamide and metformin should be avoided in patients with known renal impairment. In the insulin-treated patient the effect of insulin is prolonged and depending on carbohydrate intake, the dose of insulin may be significantly reduced. The acidosis of severe renal impairment may be mistaken for, and indeed contribute to, the problems of ketoacidosis.

The peripheral nerves

Though the number of patients with symptoms of peripheral nerve damage may be less than those with eye and kidney disease, the symptoms of neuropathy should not be under-estimated because they can cause considerable distress and are not always diagnosed accurately. Three types of peripheral nerve damage are recognisable in clinical practice (Fig. 3.7). The most common is a symmetrical, sensory, polyneuropathy which is usually chronic. Motor neuropathy on the other hand is often asymmetrical and more acute in onset; varieties of mixed sensory and motor polyneuropathy occur and also paralysis of isolated nerves (a mononeuropathy).

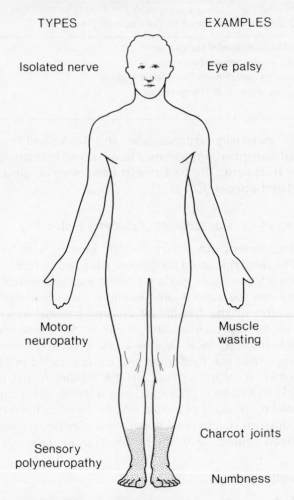

TYPES   EXAMPLES

Isolated nerve   Eye palsy

Motor neuropathy   Muscle wasting

Charcot joints

Sensory polyneuropathy

Numbness

Figure 3.7 Peripheral nerve problems in diabetes.

The typical diabetic peripheral neuropathy is a symmetrical, sensory polyneuropathy mainly affecting the lower limbs. Frequently it is asymptomatic, but when symptoms arise, numbness, tingling paraesthesia and altered sensation are noted in the feet and legs. It is often described as walking on cotton wool. Pain may be a troublesome feature, especially at night. On testing it is found that the loss of sensation occurs in a stocking distribution. Some degree of distal weakness may be present, especially in the small muscles of the foot, resulting in a claw foot deformity. In severe cases with loss of pain sensation, there is a risk of pressure and traumatic ulceration on the feet leading in the long-term to disorganised (Charcot) joints. Patients with sensory symptoms usually develop them slowly but occasionally a more acute form of polyneuropathy can occur within a few weeks of starting treatment of diabetes.

Diabetic amyotrophy is a painful motor neuropathy clinically seen as an asymmetrical muscle weakness and wasting, occurring characteristically in the thigh but it may also affect the shoulder and arm. It is often very painful, but not associated with any objective sensory loss. It usually occurs in middle-aged or elderly patients in whom it may be severe enough to make walking or even standing difficult.

Isolated nerve lesions are another separate form of neuropathy. Acute paralysis of a cranial nerve may occur abruptly. It is most commonly seen in the third and sixth nerves supplying the external eye muscles. Isolated peripheral nerve lesions can also occur, for example the ulnar and radial nerves in the arm and the femoral, sciatic and lateral (peroneal) nerves in the leg. A lesion of such a nerve is unrelated to signs of peripheral sensory polyneuropathy. Diabetic neuropathy may make a peripheral nerve more vulnerable to other injuries, though it would be difficult to prove that compression of the median nerve in the carpal tunnel at the wrist, or the sciatic nerve from a spinal disc protrusion, was any more common in diabetes.

Treatment of neuropathy

A number of different treatments have been attempted to alleviate or reverse the nerve damage. All clinicians would advise the best control possible of diabetes. This may mean starting insulin therapy, changing to twice or more daily insulin injections, or considering the use of subcutaneous infusions of insulin even though other features or poor control are not present. Any additional treatment must be assessed knowing the natural history of peripheral nerve damage. Diabetic amyotrophy tends to make a slow, full or partial recovery over several months. Isolated nerve lesions will also recover spontaneously over two to three months. The symptoms of the more common polyneuropathy may be helped by optimum diabetic control but it is not usual to show significant improvement in nerve conduction measurements, though the more acute form occurring in the initial phase of diabetic treatment usually recovers completely. The relief of symptoms of polyneuropathy may be difficult if simple analgesia is not effective and dependence on stronger analgesics is to be avoided. Nefopam is a relatively new analgesic which is not related to the narcotic agents and does not cause habituation. Drugs such as carbamazepine and phenytoin that have no marked general analgesic effect may be of value in suppressing the pain.

Autonomic neuropathy

The autonomic nervous system controls the activities of the heart, blood vessels, gut, glands and smooth muscle throughout the body. It is divided into the sympathetic and parasympathetic systems which tend to produce opposite effects on those organs which they both supply.

Damage to the nerves of the parasympathetic and sympathetic nervous system (Fig. 3.8) probably occurs at the same time as damage to the peripheral nerves. Clinical features of autonomic neuropathy are noted in Table 3.8.

Postural hypotension can be a serious symptom leading to dizziness on standing and even to syncope. Such symptoms may be confused with hypoglycaemic reactions or cerebral ischaemic attacks. Probably the simplest test of autonomic function is to measure blood pressure lying and one minute after standing up. A fall in systolic blood pressure of 10 mm mercury or less is normal and a fall of 30 mm or more is clearly abnormal. The fall in blood pressure can vary during the day and may be related to time of insulin injection.

Table 3.8 Clinical features of autonomic neuropathy

Postural hypotension
Gastric symptoms
Hypoglycaemic unawareness
Intermittent diarrhoea
Bladder atony
Impotence

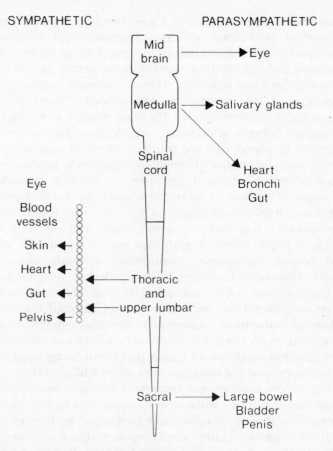

Figure 3.8 The autonomic nervous system.

Cardiac denervation has been studied in detail and shown initially to be mainly affecting the parasympathetic system (vagus nerve). This causes a rapid heart rate which is fixed, which does not alter with respiration or posture. This has been used for a number of simple non-invasive tests of autonomic function. The variation of heart rate is usually measured as the beat to beat or R–R interval on the ECG recording. The most sensitive test is to measure the beat to beat variation while the subject breathes deeply. When there is normal variation in heart rate with deep breathing, autonomic neuropathy is virtually excluded. The clinical importance of cardiac denervation is that cardiorespiratory arrest and sudden unexplained deaths occur in these patients. Unawareness of hypoglycaemia is another potentially serious consequence of autonomic neuropathy. Of the various disturbances of gastrointestinal function, diabetic diarrhoea and diabetic gastric paresis have attracted the most attention. There is delayed emptying and dilatation of the stomach despite a widely open pylorus (gastroparesis diabeticorum). Anorexia, nausea, vomiting or a persistent fullness after meals usually develop insidiously. Irregular emptying of food into the intestine may result in erratic diabetic control. Though constipation is probably the most common intestinal symptom of diabetic autonomic neuropathy it tends to be overshadowed by the problem of diarrhoea. Intermittent attacks of diarrhoea with watery stools may last for a few hours to several weeks and are frequently worse at night. When steatorrhoea occurs it is usually mild, and severe continuous steatorrhoea suggests coexisting coeliac disease or carcinoma of the pancreas. Another point to bear in mind is that diarrhoea is a relatively common side effect in patients on metformin but not through the mechanism of autonomic neuropathy. Probably several factors contribute to produce the diarrhoea of autonomic neuropathy with delayed small bowel transit which encourages bacterial colonisation and gut irritation from altered bile acids.

The urinary bladder may become denervated resulting in a large atonic bladder without any obstruction to the bladder outlet. The mixing of urine over prolonged periods of time with incomplete bladder emptying may result in unhelpful urine tests for glucose, and diabetic control may be seriously affected if urinary tract infections supervene (Table 3.9).

Facial sweating during eating (gustatory sweating) is a normal response to highly spiced foods and occurs in some normal individuals especially after chocolate or cheese. Some diabetic patients have drenching facial sweats at mealtimes, a few seconds after starting to chew tasty foodstuffs, such as cheese,

Table 3.9 Autonomic neuropathy: effects on diabetic management

Altered hypoglycaemic reactions
Erratic diabetic control
Erroneous urine test results
Difficulty in dilating the pupil
Cardio-respiratory arrest

chocolate, alcohol, pickles and others. Other abnormalities of sweating include decreased sweating over the lower half of the body and this sometimes causes heat intolerance with profuse sweating over the head and upper trunk which is unrelated to eating. The pupil can also be affected by autonomic neuropathy. It is often abnormal in patients who have had diabetes for many years. There is a poor reaction to some mydriatics and in long-term diabetes the pupil tends to be small due to reduced sympathetic activity altering the balance towards parasympathetic dominance. There is also a reduction in the spontaneous variations in size. The actual iris may become involved in the microvascular disease with the proliferation of new vessels (rubeosis iridis) and eventual scarring, adhesions and atrophy.

Erectile impotence in men occurs between two and five times more commonly in diabetic patients than in men in the same age in the general population. Various causes have been suggested, including autonomic neuropathy. Many impotent diabetic men have no other clinical features of autonomic neuropathy and normal cardiovascular reflexes. In a few of these patients other evidence of autonomic neuropathy is present or will appear later in follow-up, suggesting that impotence can be an early clinical feature of autonomic nerve damage. In most patients, however, the actual cause of the impotence is not known and could be due to vessel or nerve disease. Unfortunately no form of treatment is successful for long established impotence.

Treatment of autonomic neuropathy

The outlook for patients with autonomic neuropathy is poor. Of the causes of death, half are due to microvascular disease. There are a number of unexplained sudden deaths in this group. Cardiorespiratory arrests occur in patients undergoing anaesthesia, or are associated with a chest infection or heart failure, and there may in fact be a central brain stem abnormality. Hypoglycaemic unawareness can be fatal. Therefore, care is required in the monitoring of such patients both for diabetic control and during operation or chest infections. Simple measures such as codeine, diphenoxylate or loperamide to reduce bowel motility may be sufficient to control mild and infrequent attacks of diarrhoea. For more severe diarrhoea courses of a broad spectrum antibiotic may be helpful. Gastric paresis may be another symptom that is difficult to treat. Regular small meals may help and metoclopramide may be tried to improve gastric emptying. Surgical drainage operations are of no benefit.

The large blood vessels

a. Peripheral vascular disease

Diabetes is definitely linked to the problem of atherosclerosis of the arterial supply to the legs. Gangrene occurs about five times more frequently in the diabetic in comparison with the non-diabetic population in western societies. Of the many causes and associated factors of atherosclerosis smoking appears to be particularly important for peripheral vascular disease. The disease in the diabetic patient is similar to the non-diabetic except when it tends to be more diffuse and affect the smaller arteries below the knee. The clinical features will depend upon the severity of distribution of the disease and may be modified if significant peripheral neuropathy is also present. The most common symptom is intermittent claudication with ischaemic pain in the calf, thigh or buttock areas occurring on exercise. Other symptoms include cold feet, poor healing and in patients with more proximal disease, impotence. More serious symptoms include pain at rest, ischaemic foot ulcers and gangrene. The recognition of ischaemic changes is a vital part of the management of the diabetic foot (see below). The skin becomes thin (atrophic), shiny and cool and the peripheral arteries will not be palpable, and capillary filling slow after the skin has been pressed. The overall colour of the skin may be red, pale or cyanosed. A blanching will occur on elevating the ischaemic leg to 45° for 1 to 2 minutes. Ischaemic ulcers are usually distal involving the toes, the distal part of the foot, or pressure areas around the big and little toes and the ankle.

It is rarely necessary to perform arteriography to confirm peripheral vascular disease except when it is thought that a block may have occurred in an iliac or femoral artery in a

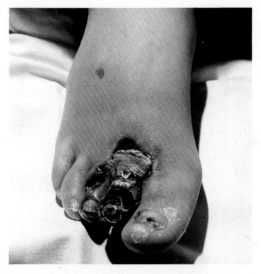

Colour Plate 3:
Gangrene of the second and third toes due to ischaemia. Note also dystrophic nails, the scaly skin of the great toe, and the redness of the dorsum of the foot.

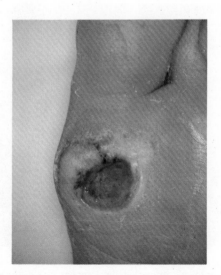

Colour Plate 4:
Ulceration at the base of the great toe. Typically there is a deep 'punched-out' ulcer at a pressure point. Loss of sensation, infection, and lack of foot care all contribute to these lesions.

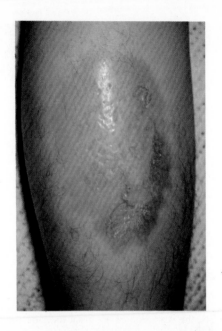

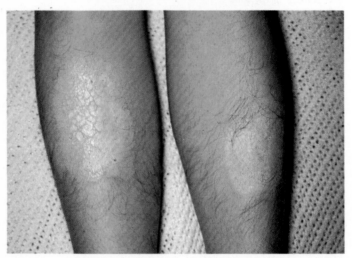

Colour Plate 5:
Necrobiosis lipoidica – Above – typical appearance of the skin.
Bottom – disguised with a cover-up cream.

younger patient where surgical correction is a possibility. The Doppler ultrasound detector is useful in giving a more accurate assessment of the peripheral pulses.

In the management of peripheral vascular disease peripheral vasodilators are often tried but with little proven effect. It is reasonable to avoid vasoconstrictor drugs, however, such as propranolol. In peripheral vascular disease when rest pain has occurred adequate analgesics are important and severe pain should not be so prolonged as to result in phantom limb phenomenon when amputation is done. Conservative surgery is not usually done for ischaemic change, though occasionally lumbar sympathectomy is useful. Below or above knee amputation is often necessary, as it is only rarely possible to excise small local areas of gangrene. Gangrene of an individual toe can be left untreated to amputate itself provided the toe remains dry and uninfected.

b. Coronary artery disease

Diabetes increases the risk of developing coronary artery disease, especially in women. By itself diabetes is not a very high risk factor, but will be additional to the effects of other factors present, such as a strong family history of coronary artery disease, smoking, hypertension and hyperlipidaemia. There is also concern that oral contraceptives may be aggravating diabetes and contributing to premature vascular disease in women. The clinical features of angina and most myocardial infarctions occurring in patients with known diabetes are similar to non-diabetic patients. Myocardial infarction, however, may be silent—that is, free of acute pain—but discovered either because of deterioration in diabetic control, the appearance of arrhythmias or cardiac failure, or on routine electrocardiography. Silent myocardial infarctions also occur in the non-diabetic population. The consequences of myocardial infarction are much more serious in the diabetic compared with the non-diabetic patient. The overall mortality of tablet and insulin-treated patients is doubled compared with non-diabetics at approximately 40 per cent. Diet-treated patients are similar to the non-diabetic patient.

After a myocardial infarction the occurrence of congestive

cardiac failure is greater in diabetic than in non-diabetic patients. The increased risk of congestive failure, however, is not explained by coexisting overt coronary disease and is largely confined to the insulin-treated patients. Diabetic patients are more prone than non-diabetics to recurrence of myocardial infarction and myocardial rupture.

The additional problems for diabetic patients with myocardial infarction may be due to some disease of the myocardium resulting from microvascular as well as macrovascular processes. It has also been suggested that collateral development may be impaired or a direct metabolic abnormality affects myocardial function. It is hardly surprising to find that the long-term outlook of a diabetic patient with their first myocardial infarction is poor compared with a non-diabetic patient. A diabetic patient has about a 20 per cent chance of being alive five years later, compared with a 50–70 per cent 5-year survival in non-diabetics.

Treatment of coronary artery disease. The management of myocardial infarction, angina and cardiac failure is similar to that in the non-diabetic patient with additional care in the use of diuretics and beta-blockade drugs.

Problems in the management of diabetic patients (Ch. 4). Myocardial infarction causes a similar metabolic stress as a surgical operation and will result in deterioration in diabetic control (Table 3.10). Indeed this may be the first time that diabetes is diagnosed. The patient with known diabetes controlled on diet alone or oral hypoglycaemic drugs will often require insulin therapy during the first week after a myocardial infarction. Later requirements may depend on the extent of the infarction limiting patient activity. Angina itself does not affect diabetic control but in the insulin-treated patient care should be taken to warn the patient who is given a beta-blockade drug such as propranolol, that hypoglycaemic reac-

Table 3.10 Ischaemic heart disease: effects on diabetic management

Avoid hypoglycaemia	
Diabetic control may be altered by:	blood glucose trend
myocardial infarction	↑
congestive cardiac failure	↓
diuretic therapy	↑

tions may be altered. There is also some concern that a severe hypoglycaemic attack itself may precipitate a myocardial infarction in a patient who already has some coronary artery disease so that very low blood glucose control is usually avoided. The treatment of congestive cardiac failure is similar as in a non-diabetic patient, although loss of appetite and hepatic congestion may result in lower blood glucose levels and a reduction in hypoglycaemic therapy. This may be balanced by the effect of diuretic therapy inhibiting insulin release and increasing blood glucose levels. Diuretics will not have any effect on diabetic control in the insulin-deficient patient who is already on insulin treatment.

c. Cerebral arterial disease

Strokes are about twice as common in diabetic patients than in non-diabetics. Of all the risk factors of macrovascular disease, hypertension is the most important factor associated with strokes. The management of a transient ischaemic attack and a fully established stroke in the diabetic patient is no different from the non-diabetic, although the outlook is somewhat worse with 50 per cent of patients dying within a year.

The importance of strokes in a patient with treated diabetes is that hypoglycaemia may present as a transient ischaemic attack or what appears to be a fully established stroke. On treatment of the hypoglycaemia the stroke will recover. Transient ischaemic attacks may also result from postural hypotension (see above).

The diabetic foot (Colour plates 3 and 4)

The foot of a diabetic patient is a special problem resulting in a variety of lesions ranging from minor callous formation to fulminating infection and gangrene. An established lesion may cause great suffering, involving long admissions to hospital and the need for much nursing and medical care. Greater understanding of the pathology of the diabetic foot should lead to greater awareness by the patient, and all who care for diabetic patients, of the vital importance of prevention and early treatment of foot problems.

The diabetic foot may show changes entirely due to either

ischaemia or peripheral neuropathy. Many problems though are due to a combination of ischaemia and peripheral neuropathy with superadded infection. In an individual patient, management depends on an accurate assessment on whether it is primarily a problem of ischaemia or neuropathy. Ischaemia in a foot may arise in several ways. Thrombotic occlusion of a large vessel will result in gangrene of a large segment of the leg. More peripheral arterial occlusions will result in small and patchy areas of gangrene in the foot and toes. Ischaemia of a single toe or the adjacent sides of two toes may be due to embolic fragments becoming detached from a patch of atheroma in the aorta or other large vessel and lodging in a small artery in the foot. Infection in a toe may also precipitate local gangrene. It is also possible that poor perfusion of the skin could result from microvascular disease with capillary closure and arteriovenous shunting.

Neuropathy results in another sequence of foot problems. Loss of pain and temperature sensation means that mechanical trauma and injury from chemicals and excessive heat or cold go unnoticed. Foot deformities also occur, the more common being a claw foot due to muscle weakness. Excessive pressure under the heads of the metatarsals and over the top of the toes in such a deformed foot results in extensive callous formation: later, painless ulceration may follow. Foot deformities may also occur following surgery and when loss of sensation results in damaged (Charcot) joints.

Some of the important distinguishing features are noted in Table 3.11. The ischaemic foot is recognised by being painful, feeling cold, with skin that is reddened with the foot lowered and blanched on elevation. The skin and the subcutaneous fatty tissues may be atrophic and ulceration and gangrene may be present. In contrast the neuropathic foot may be surprisingly pain free, feels warm and the skin may be thickened with callous formation, especially around ulceration at pressure points.

Ulceration in the diabetic foot may occur secondary to ischaemia or to neuropathy. An amazing amount of traumatic damage can occur without being recognised in the neuropathic foot. Some ulcers may occur secondarily to blister formation. Two types of blister occur in the diabetic foot; an acute superficial blister which heals rapidly and a deeper

Table 3.11 Clinical signs in the diabetic foot

	Ischaemia	Neuropathy
Pain	Considerable	Relatively free
Deformity	Nil	May be present
Skin	Thin Rubor on dependency Blanches on elevation	Often callous formation Normal colour
Temperature	Feels cold	Feels normal
Subcutaneous tissues	Atrophic	Normal
Peripheral pulses	Absent	Present

haemorrhagic type which may lead to ulceration. The precise mechanisms for these blisters is not known, but it is possible that the deeper ones are caused by a shear strain on the skin.

Infection adds enormously to the problems of the diabetic foot. Infection may arise through poor hygiene, paronychia, fungal disease and through any breach or breakdown of the skin. *Staphylococcus aureus* is an important infecting organism in many foot lesions but mixed infections can occur. Some of the micro-organisms present may be contaminants from the surrounding skin. The progression of infection in the diabetic foot may be alarmingly swift with some staphylococci and streptococci sepsis. Gas may form in the tissues and may be detected either clinically by the feeling of crepitus or on x-ray, and does not mean that gas gangrene has occurred. Chronic foot sepsis may become very deep-seated with involvement of underlying bones and joints when it cannot usually be eradicated by medical measures.

Management

Prevention of foot problems is an essential part of the education and re-education of the diabetic patient, particularly those in whom there is already evidence of peripheral vascular or nerve disease. An example should be set by examining feet carefully in the clinic with instruction to the patient to examine feet regularly at home. Someone else may need to do this for the elderly and those with poor vision. Daily washing with thorough drying and the wearing of clean stockings are important. Patients should be warned not to walk barefooted and to avoid using hot water bottles, hot soaks, strong disinfectants, chemicals and corn cures, and should be careful when applying and removing adhesive plasters. Care should be taken to find good fitting shoes, and to break-in new shoes gradually. Any difficult nail cutting and any treatment required for corns and callosities should be left to a chiropodist.

The value of specific preventive measures to combat major ischaemia of the legs in diabetes is more difficult to prove. Avoidance of cigarette smoking is probably important. Specific medical measures to aid the circulation in established peripheral vascular disease are also of no proven value, though vasodilator drugs are often prescribed. Lumbar sympathectomy operations are occasionally undertaken in an attempt to improve skin blood flow. Reconstructive arterial surgery can sometimes be undertaken in the relatively young diabetic patient whose peripheral vascular disease is largely proximal.

The treatment of a major diabetic foot problem is best undertaken jointly by the physician and an orthopaedic surgeon. Rest and control of infection are basic. Ischaemic lesions will heal poorly or not at all and local surgery is rarely successful. The outlook for an ischaemic foot is much worse than a primary neuropathic lesion. A neuropathic ulcer may heal if infection is controlled, and local amputation is usually successful in removing grossly damaged tissue. Foot ulcers should be cleaned with antiseptics, such as sodium hypochlorite, and covered with non-adhesive dressings. Debridement of overhanging ulcer edges and deep necrotic slough will aid healing. Systemic antibiotics will be needed if there is severe sepsis and cellulitis in the foot, and adequate local drainage must be ensured if the presence of pus is suspected.

Amputation is often required for ischaemic lesions and often at the below knee level. Small areas of dry painless gangrene, as in an individual toe, may be left without operation. Amputation is required later in the management of neuropathic foot problems and often a ray excision of a toe may be all that is required. While attention is being paid to the diabetic foot problem on one side, the health and safety of the foot on the other side must not be neglected. The results after amputation will depend not only on the satisfactory healing of the operation site and the fitting of a satisfactory prosthesis but also on the state of the remaining foot. The patient who has required amputation because of diabetes has a high risk, approximately 40 per cent within three years, of amputation of the second leg.

The diabetic hand

Waxy thickening of the skin in the hands, associated with pain and stiffness, has been associated with insulin-dependent diabetes. One simple method of detecting such abnormalities is to ask the patient to approximate the palmar surfaces of the interphalangeal joints of both hands tightly with the fingers spread. The frequency, significance, and cause are disputed. Different groups have reported between 8 and 32 per cent of patients affected where diabetes had been diagnosed in child-hood and adolescence. To what extent it is inherited within the families of insulin-dependent patients and whether it is related to long-term microvascular complications is unknown.

The skin

Infections of the skin including boils, carbuncles and moni-liasis (thrush) seem to occur more commonly in diabetic patients, particularly at times of poor control. It is also quite common for glycosuria to be found, and diabetes diagnosed, in patients attending with boils or carbuncles. Another group of skin changes occuring in diabetic patients is the deposition of lipid (fat) in the skin. Xanthelasma is the name for the yellow fat deposits on the eye-lids, while xanthomata may occur as fleshy tuberous growths over bony prominences.

A specific skin change occurring in diabetic patients is necrobiosis lipoidica. Usually this occurs on the front of the shins and consists of a yellowish central area surrounded by a red papular area (see Colour plate 5). It may occur before diabetes is diagnosed and once developed tends to persist although occasionally it may heal spontaneously. The lesions are unsightly and while trousers may hide the condition, young female patients may need to apply a masking cream and wear slightly heavier tights or stockings. Covermark (Stiefel) is a suit-able cream and since it comes in a variety of shades this can be matched to the patient's skin colour (Colour plate 5).

4

Caring for the diabetic patient

ORGANISATION OF DIABETIC CARE

A. OUT-PATIENT CARE

Introduction

Diabetic clinics were established soon after the introduction of insulin in 1922 and the British Diabetic Association, founded in 1934, further encouraged the setting up of such clinics when it became apparent that insulin-dependent patients required specialist care. With an increasing population, however, many of the older, hospital-based clinics have become huge, unwieldy, and logistically almost impossible to manage. This has led a number of authors to pose the question 'has the centralisation of diabetic care led to an atrophy of the necessary skills in other doctors and nurses and generated ignorance and fear of the disease?' In this chapter we shall firstly consider the functions of a diabetic clinic (Table 4.1) and the role of the nurse within the clinic (Table 4.2). A consider-able proportion of these sections apply equally whether the clinic is a hospital-based diabetic clinic or one of the alterna-tive, community-based methods of caring for the diabetic. In the second part of the chapter we shall compare the hospital-

Table 4.1 The function of the diabetic clinic

1. Diagnosis and full clinical assessment
2. Instigating treatment
3. Education of patients and staff
4. Follow-up and documentation of progress
5. Screening for complications
6. Close supervision of special groups of patients e.g. pregnant women, adolescents
7. Assessment and referral of patients with specific needs e.g. surgery, chiropody
8. Therapeutic trials
9. Research

based diabetic clinic with alternative methods of management and care and finally we will consider in-patient care of the diabetic patient.

Records

Diabetes is a chronic disorder and patients may attend a clinic for more than twenty or thirty years. During this time they may accumulate vast quantities of out-patient notes and their hospital record may include kilograms of in-patient records. It is of utmost importance, therefore, that documentation is accurate, concise and systematic, so the changes which occur from visit to visit can be readily seen. Two areas are of particular importance. Firstly, the recordings which are obtained when the patient first attends the clinic are invaluable as a baseline for comparison during follow-up. Secondly, the follow-up record should allow a ready appreciation of the patient's progress.

First attendance

When the patient first attends a diabetic clinic certain features should be carefully recorded. These include in the history, the presence of symptoms, the family history, patient's previous medical history and their continuing on other drug therapy, and in women the obstetric history. Careful documentation of the physical examination should include the detection of complications of diabetes and the presence of co-existing disease. It is important at this stage to confirm the diagnosis of diabetes. The patient's urine should be tested for glycosuria, ketonuria and proteinuria, and a blood glucose estimated. The patient's height should be measured and weight recorded and the percentage of desirable body weight obtained from tables. In children or adolescents a growth chart should be commenced at this stage.

Follow-up record

A flow chart allows for easy access to information and progress. An example of the flow chart which we use is displayed in Figure 4.1. At each visit to the clinic the patient's blood glucose is estimated and recorded on the graph. It is

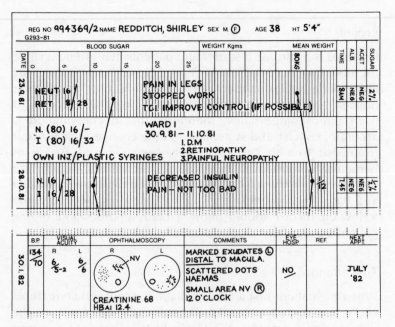

Figure 4.1 An example of a follow-up record for patients attending a diabetic clinic.

also particularly useful to record the patient's body weight in graphical form. A record is also kept of urine tests for glucose, ketones and protein. Specific examination such as visual acuity and ophthalmoscopy can be highlighted by using a rubber stamp, as can attendance at a special clinic.

Other parameters of control such as glycosylated haemoglobin, home blood glucose monitoring estimations and serum creatinine can also be recorded. It is useful to record brief details of in-patient addmissions particularly the problem for which the patient was admitted, any procedures which were carried out and the diabetic therapy at discharge, as well as any other drug therapy.

We would not pretend that our follow-up record is ideal. It is all too easy to overlook other aspects of the patient's condition, in particular which other drugs are taken, when the eyes were last looked at and when the blood pressure was last recorded.

With attendance at a clinic for thirty years or more notes may become vast and unmanageable. Computerised records would appear to be the answer. A number of clinics, notably St Thomas's Hospital and King's College Hospital, both in London, have tried such systems with variable success. Recently the Diabetes Unit in Nottingham have developed a system with which they report good results.

Other aspects of documentation

Clinic appointment cards should carry as much information as possible including blood glucose and weight at each visit and visual acuity when this is carried out. There should be a space for listing medication other than insulin or hypoglycaemic agents, e.g. diuretics, beta-blockers or corticosteroids. Ideally separate cards for those on insulin and oral hypoglycaemic agents are preferred with a different format and colour.

Of considerable importance in the hospital clinic are the letters to the primary care doctor. Communication of changes in therapy or changes in the patient's condition should be made simply and clearly. This is likely to be of increasing importance in the future in view of the similarity in names of oral hypoglycaemic agents and of insulins.

THE ROLE OF THE NURSE IN THE DIABETIC CLINIC

Nurses who work in diabetic clinics may be divided into two groups—those who fulfil their role in the out-patient clinic whenever they are needed, and those who take a lively and intensive interest in diabetic patients, not only remembering individual names and particular interests and problems, but noting almost imperceptible changes in weight or appearance which may indicate a deterioration or an improvement in a patient's condition. In this respect, the smaller community-based clinics are likely to fare better than the large hospital clinic. It should not be forgotten particularly in the large hospital clinic, just how much benefit is gained by the patients in seeing familiar faces amongst the nursing staff especially in view of patients' complaints that they rarely manage to see the same doctor twice.

The co-ordination and smooth running of a diabetic clinic is primarily the role of the clinic sister. Her enthusiasm for the task affects the attitude not only of doctors in the clinic but also of the junior nurses, and the way which she deals with ill-tempered doctors and patients will be an education for her junior nurses. She will allocate the specific nursing responsibilities within the diabetic clinic (Table 4.2).

1. Weighing patients

The accurate weighing of patients on each attendance at the clinic is of utmost importance. The nurse responsible for this should be trained in the use of desirable body weight tables and should have some appreciation of the significance of weight loss. In the over-weight patient even a small degree of

Table 4.2 Specific nursing responsibilities within the diabetic clinic

1. Weighing patients
2. Urine testing
3. Visual acuity
4. Installation of eye drops for pupil dilatation
5. Surgical dressings
6. Education of patients in urine testing or blood glucose measurement
7. Advising patients with specific problems

weight loss should meet with enthusiastic encouragement while in the older patient who is not over-weight, significant weight loss may indicate neglect, poor diabetic control, or the development of further disease. In children or adolescents, growth charts are most important and should be completed on each attendance.

2. Urine testing

Urine testing has been for many years the only method the patient had for assessing diabetic control. With the introduction of home blood glucose monitoring by the patient this situation is gradually changing. We must ask, therefore, how significant is urine testing in the diabetic clinic? After all, the patient's blood glucose will be estimated. Urine testing for glucose in the diabetic clinic remains important. Lack of correlation between blood glucose and urine glucose may alert the doctor to an abnormal renal threshold for glucose and may help to indicate a need for blood glucose monitoring in such a patient. In addition, the majority of patients will continue to monitor their diabetic control on urine tests for some time to come, and testing in the clinic helps reinforce the importance of this concept. The reverse situation can often be seen in the indifference with which some doctors discuss the ticks or crosses in a much-thumbed urine testing record book and this should be strongly discouraged. Alternating enthusiasm and indifference displayed by medical and nursing staff can only lead to confusion and apathy on the part of the patient.

Of equal importance to testing for glucose in the urine is the testing for ketones and for albumin. The presence of ketonuria may well indicate poor diabetic control but may also suggest that the patient is starving in an attempt to improve their blood glucose reading. One of the earliest signs of the development of kidney damage from diabetes is intermittent proteinuria and careful documentation of this may alert the doctor to the development of this problem.

Urine testing equipment

Before the introduction of Clinitest, patients and hospital staff used Benedict's solution to assess urine glucose. The hazards associated with boiling a mixture of Benedict's solution and urine in a test-tube over a spirit lamp can be imagined. Clinitest simplified urine testing, greatly increased its accuracy, and certainly made it safer. Diastix has simplified the procedure even further and made urine testing aesthetically more acceptable to many people and to the nurse faced with the testing of a hundred urines in a diabetic clinic. The range of Diastix is limited from negative to 2 per cent in contrast to Clinitest where, with manipulation of the number of drops of urine in the test-tube, 5 and 10 per cent glycosuria can be estimated. It is most important to realise that the enzyme reaction of Diastix can be suppressed by the presence of large amounts of ketones. For this reason many paediatricians prefer Clinitest to Diastix and patients at risk of ketonuria or ketoacidosis should be supplied with Ketostix or Ketodiastix. When educating the patient in the use of these stix a clear explanation of the effect of ketones on the colour development of Diastix should be made. For the vast majority of patients, however, Diastix are satisfactory and can be recommended for ease of use and interpretation. Timing is important in all urine testing and a stop-clock or watch is an important piece of clinic equipment.

Ketodiastix and Albustix are ideal for use in large diabetic clinics. The time saved in cleaning up as well as the speed with which tests can be carried out is no mean consideration when a hundred or more urines have to be tested.

3. Visual acuity

Visual acuity or accuracy of vision, is the ability of each eye to perceive the shape and form of objects in direct vision. In 1862 Snellen introduced test charts which have undergone little change since that time. Snellen's test type consists of horizontal rows of letters graduated in size. Each row is numbered from the top to the bottom, 60, 36, 24, 18, 12, 9, 6, 5, 4. The numbers indicate the distance in metres at which a person with normal vision can see each row. Thus the patient with normal vision should be able to read the sixth row at six metres.

There is a British Standard Specification for test charts (BS4274) with recommendations for positioning and illumination. Ideally, Snellen's test type should be internally illuminated, but for the external illuminated chart various methods of lighting are suggested. Information can be obtained from the British Standards Institution, Newton House, 101/113 Pentonville Road, London N1.

Procedure

Stand the patient at a distance of six metres from the chart. One eye is covered completely using an opaque card and not the hand. Patients with distance glasses should wear them for the test. The patient is asked to read from the top line downwards—note the last line which is read correctly. Normal vision is expressed as 6/6; with good illumination 6/5 is usual. If the patient cannot read the top letter at 6 metres he is asked to approach the chart until able to read it. If this is at 4 metres the visual acuity is recorded as 4/60. If the vision is less than 2 metres (2/60) the patient is asked to count fingers at different distances or hand movements and, finally, if unable to do any of this the patient's ability to perceive light is noted.

Young children and illiterate patients can be tested using the E test, Landolt's broken ring or picture charts. The E test is

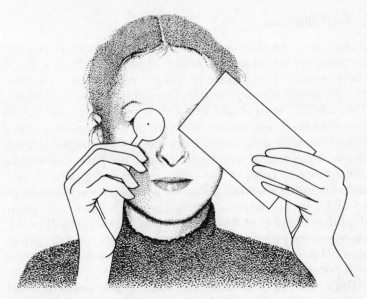

Figure 4.2 Measuring visual acuity using a pin-hole.

similar to the Snellen's test type but all the letters are Es facing in different directions. A cut-out letter E is given to the patient who turns the letter in the position indicated on the chart. Alternatively a cube can be used with different sized Es on each side. Another test for children or other patients who are not familiar with English (Roman) capital letters is the Sheridan Gardiner test. The patient holds a key card and indicates which letter is being shown by the examiner standing at a distance of 6 metres from the patient.

If the visual acuity is worse than 6/9 a pin-hole should be used (Fig. 4.2). Pin-holes reduce most visual defects due to the changes in refraction of the lens. This can easily be verified by anyone who wears distance glasses. Without these spectacles the chart may be impossible to read. The use of the pin-hole produces an amazing clarity. Since refraction changes may be associated with hyperglycaemia the use of the pin-hole helps to differentiate this benign transitory symptom from potentially serious pathology. The importance of a deteriotating visual acuity cannot be over-emphasised. It may indicate progression of diabetic retinopathy and alert the doctor to the need for careful ophthalmoscopy.

4. Pupil dilatation

Dilatation of the pupil is essential for a full ophthalmoscopic examination including the retina, choroid, and optic discs. There is often a reluctance to dilate a pupil since installation of a mydriatic may precipitate glaucoma in some individuals. It should be emphasised that this is extremely rare but all nurses in the clinic should be aware of it and patients with a history of glaucoma should not have their pupils dilated. Ideally, if ophthalmoscopy is anticipated the patient should be advised not to drive to the clinic and to bring dark glasses. Recommended mydriatics include Mydrilate (cyclopentolate) 0.5 to 1 per cent, Mydriacyl (tropicamide) 0.5 per cent, phenylephrine 10 per cent. These drops may act for up to 24 hours, however, the effect can be reversed by installation of pilocarpine 2–4 per cent drops. Tropicamide does not require reversal with pilocarpine since its effect is short-lived.

The clinic nurse should have some appreciation of which patients will need careful eye examination. For this purpose patients are grouped according to age at diagnosis. Patients under 20 years of age at diagnosis should have careful examination at five and ten years after diagnosis and then yearly. In addition, the fundus should be carefully examined in the following circumstances:

a. when a patient becomes pregnant and four months after delivery
b. when the contraceptive pill is prescribed
c. if other diabetic complications develop
d. at times of poor control

Patients who are aged over 40 years at diagnosis should have their visual acuity checked each year. Careful ophthalmoscopy should be performed every five years or if there is impairment of visual acuity. Patients aged 20–39 years at diagnosis are examined according to their treatment—insulin-dependent patients as for those aged 20 years at diagnosis, and non-insulin-dependent patients as for those over 40 years at diagnosis.

The management of such a programme is no simple task. It calls for close collaboration between medical, nursing and clerical staff. The need for screening for diabetic retinopathy is of paramount importance and the long-term benefits for patients cannot be denied. Nursing staff in a community-based clinic should not be afraid to insist or nag the doctor into careful examination of the patient's eyes. The lack of confidence in the enthusiasm or ability of the family practitioner to examine the eyes is perhaps the single most important reason why few patients are discharged from a hospital clinic. This has led to numerous suggestions for alternative methods of screening utilising ophthalmic opticians or training nurses for the task. When this is suggested, we must ask the question 'What exactly are we doing in our diabetic clinics that we do not have time to carefully look at the patients' eyes?'

5. Surgical dressings

The dressing of wounds is an integral part of the training of all nursing staff. The commonest wound encountered in a diabetic clinic is ulceration of the feet. Elsewhere in this volume we have stressed the importance of foot care. The nurse in the clinic will often be called upon to remove dressings which have previously been applied. Great care must be taken while doing this. It must be remembered that diabetic neuropathy decreases pain sensation in the foot and it is possible to carelessly remove large areas of skin without the patient appreciating pain. Similarly, in the presence of peripheral vascular disease a carelessly applied or removed dressing may do damage which will take many months to heal.

The nurse should be clear in her own mind of the clinic policy with respect to ulceration of the feet. The dressing applied most frequently in our own clinic is a dry dressing following a wash with eusol. In particular, local antibiotic creams, ointments, or powders have not been convincingly demonstrated to be of benefit.

While removing and applying dressings is an ideal time for the nurse to get over to the patient some basic ideas on footcare. It is also a suitable time to assess that chiropody may be of benefit and, in helping the elderly patient to remove shoes or put on shoes, the nurse may spot ill-fitting footwear and advise the patient accordingly.

6. Teaching patients

Teaching patients to test urine or to carry out blood glucose estimation is far from difficult. Traditionally, this task falls to the nurse on the ward or in the clinic and the sheer mechanics of how to test and how to record results can easily be taught to the majority of patients. What is far less easy is to convey to the patient what action should be taken in response to the results obtained. For many years patients have recorded their urine tests with almost religious fervour carrying them by the bookful to their local clinic. The change to home blood glucose monitoring has been welcomed by many patients, but the crucial factor in both these exercises is not the testing of the urine or blood and the recording of the results but how the patient uses those results. This will mean that patients have to be given sound advice on how to change their insulins in response to particular patterns of results obtained. At present by law in the U.K. nurses are prevented from changing insulin doses and any deviation from this must depend on mutual trust and faith of doctors and nurses locally. If it is to remain the responsibility of the doctor to advise the patient on how to alter their therapy in response to blood glucose measurements at home, then the nurse should ensure that details of the technique and advice on therapy modification are given together and form part of an educational programme.

7. Advising patients with any problems

It is a well-known fact that patients will often confide in a nurse information which they would not share with the doctor. This may be particularly about their diabetes and aspects of diabetic control including things which they regard as too trivial to bother the doctor with. It may also include particular problems they are encountering at home with respect to family or job or social circumstances. Patients should be encouraged to share this information and be prompted by the nurse to inform the doctor where it is felt appropriate. The nurse must be aware, however, that while most patients are reasonable people, as with all walks of life occasional difficult personalities are encountered. Such a patient in the clinic may make a beeline for a particular nurse to confide the latest episode of a saga. They may also make considerable demands upon the time of specialist nurses. The professional must be aware of the point where further investment of time in a particular patient does not produce further benefits in terms of educational treatment. This is one of the most difficult lessons for a nurse to learn but the precious resource of a nurse's time available for education of patients must not be wasted on those patients who are rather more interested in the manipulation of the relationship.

Fortunately such patients are few and far between. The majority of patients are reasonable patients who wish for advice on specific points and have concerns which are important to them no matter how trivial they seem to professional staff with whom they come into contact.

THE COMMUNITY NURSE ATTACHED TO THE HOSPITAL CLINIC

At this point it would be pertinent to consider the role of a very important nurse attached to the hospital clinic. This is the community nurse who spends her time working outside the hospital clinic attached to community services. The great asset of the holder of such a post is that by visiting the local hospital clinic, problems can be identified which may be pursued into the patient's home. Referral of patients to her may be by the doctor or dietician, or by the clinic nurse who may feel that they have been presented with a problem by a patient and not managed to to resolve it. A home visit can then be arranged following which, at the next diabetic clinic, further discussion can take place and suggestions for resolving the problem.

The role of this nurse may best be shown by two examples taken from our own clinic.

Mrs Christopher is a 48-year-old blind widow whose diabetes is normally well controlled. For no apparent reason she began to experience hypoglycaemic attacks and indeed attended the casualty department of the hospital three times in one month. The clinic sister felt that this change in her control was associated with some worries which she had, yet the patient was insistent that this was not so and she was all right.

The assistance of the community nurse was sought and she subsequently visited the patient at home. She found her to have a very pleasant 16-year-old son and the pair of them lived in their 1930 semi-detached home which she owned having paid off the mortgage with money she received at the time of her husband's death twelve years previously. In the course of conversation it transpired that the next door neighbour's house had recently been electrically rewired. The patient has sought an estimate for rewiring her own house and found that this came to just under £200. This was a sum which was beyond her means as her son had recently left school and was working as an apprentice 25 miles away. His fares to and from his work took up a considerable amount of his pay to the extent that his mother was worse off than when her son had been at school.

The problem was compounded by her being told that the electrical wiring of her house was totally inadequate and that she was sitting on a 'time bomb'.

The social services were unable to help her as she owned her own home and in turn she was unable to see any way out of her problem until she had saved the money. In view of this it seemed likely that her food intake was being restricted in an attempt to save.

The community nurse had clearly identified the problem and she now turned to authorities from whom she felt help might be obtained. In a very short time the British Diabetic Association and the Royal National Institute for the Blind had been contacted and indicated that they were willing to pay the sum to have the house rewired. The outcome for the patient was that an apparently unstable diabetic was returned to her former self.

This case history illustrates not only the value of the community nurse in identifying problems not readily accessible to the clinic staff, but also accentuates the important point that when a previously stable diabetic patient begins experiencing hypoglycaemia every attempt should be made to identify the cause of this change.

Mr Watson is a 70-year-old diabetic patient who recently complained of increasing hypoglcaemic attacks occurring during the night. On many occasions he was seen by the dietician who went over his diet with him and by the doctor who repeatedly altered his insulin dose. This did not lead to a change in his condition. Eventually, he was referred to the community nurse by the dietician who made the request for the nurse to see the patient's wife as she never accompanied him to the diabetic clinic.

At the home visit the old gentleman was out shopping and the nurse was able to listen to the wife's long tale about how he would never let her come to the clinic as she would only grumble too much about the trouble he caused her during the night. Most nights she would have to knock on the wall to wake up her next door neighbours who would then come to help treat his hypoglycaemic attack. During his hypoglycaemic attacks he would become disorientated and aggressive and refuse to take glucose. Having sufficiently roused him she would then have to change the bed linen and his pyjamas because of his sweating and not surprisingly, she grumbled to him about the extra work, her lack of sleep, and the worry that they were causing their 'golden' neighbours. When Mr Watson returned the nurse talked about his diet, his insulin technique and his eyesight, plus all the customary discussion of regular meals and bed-time snacks, and all seemed satisfactory. Eventually he was asked at what time did he give his insulin. 'Before I retired' he said 'I used to give it at 5.30, but lately I have been leaving it a little later to 6.00 or 6.30'. The nurse suggested that maybe these times were a little bit early now that he had retired and had no need to go to work. It was not until this point that it was discovered that he was talking about the evening and not the morning. It transpired that during his working life he had worked permanent night-shift. On leaving work at the age of 65 years it had not occurred to him to change the time of his injection and he had persisted with his evening injection for 5 years.

These tales are neither fictitious nor uncommon. The situations arise from the patient not wishing to trouble the doctor or the nurse in the clinic with his or her problems. We all must realise that control of a patient's diabetes is a complicated process which stretches far from the situation in the clinic. Funding authorities have been slow in realising the benefits of community nurses, trained in and assigned to the care of the diabetic. In their terms the cost of ambulance transport to casualty depertments or repeated visits to diabetic clinics should be weighed against the cost of adequate staff to enter the patient's home. In our terms the disruption of repeated hypoglycaemia and the loss of confidence which this engenders must be a major concern in our teaching of patients to live 'normal' lives. The community nurse attached to the hospital clinic contributes significantly to this goal.

THE ROLE OF THE DIETICIAN

Diet is almost synonymous with diabetes. Medication may vary but diet remains at the core of diabetic management. The dietician therefore has a key position in the diabetes care team. The vast majority of dieticians are hospital based and form part of the clinic team. Some health districts have community dieticians who are able to visit patients in their own homes ostensibly to make a more realistic assessment of the patient's eating patterns. This would appear to be the ideal arrangement but not enough hard data have been compiled to prove the cost-effectiveness of this approach. The peripatetic dietician may travel many miles to see two or three patients in one morning or afternoon, whereas twice or three times as many patients could be seen in a dietetic out-patient clinic; but the proof of the pudding is in the eating and the proof of effective dietary education is in the long-term compliance of the patient.

Assessing the dietary/nutritional needs of the patient will depend on many factors including type of diabetes and medication, pre-existing eating patterns, body weight, age, lifestyle, employment if any, income, sporting activities, ethnic groups, intellect and common sense and so on.

A dietary history is essential and the template on which a diabetic diet is based, for unless the patient's diet is bizzare or unsatisfactory from the nutritional point of view, the pre-existing dietary intake is modified and adapted with, it is hoped, the minimum amount of disruption and change. The exception is the obese patient who must reduce his or her total calorific intake. Such a patient presents the dietician with a great challenge and a problem which may prove insoluble. The dietician is both teacher and mentor and must have the ability to influence, to encourage without being too didactic or authoritarian.

Most dietary education is carried out on a one to one basis using the spoken and written word. There appears to be a dearth of well-illustrated and interestingly produced patient literature for the dietician to use. Food models are an excellent way to present an entire meal and can be used in a clinic setting with the minimum amount of fuss. The models are expensive but very realistic and durable. Many dieticians have produced their own teaching aids and those working under ideal conditions actually prepare demonstration meals with the patient in a kitchen setting.

Patient education and the production of audio-visual aids is discussed in Chapter 5. Unfortunately, most dietary education takes place at or around the time of diagnosis when the patient is the least receptive and is unable to comprehend what is being said to him. Most centres arrange for a dietary follow-up but all too often the one and only encounter the non-insulin-dependent diabetic has with a dietician is at diagnosis. Informal group sessions would appear to be beneficial for both insulin-dependent and non-insulin-dependent patients and would augment the individual teaching and make optimum use of finite resources.

The dietary recommendation introduced in 1981 encourages a high-fibre, high carbohydrate diet with reduced fat and protein intake. On the 4th November 1982 the British Diabetic Association issued its new dietary recommendations for diabetics in the 80s. The original recommendations have been modified and the British Diabetic Association have produced new guidelines. There are slide/tape programmes and a new cook book showing the practical application of the new diet but in spite of this plethora of dietary information, we still lack simply written, clearly illustrated leaflets giving the basic information on these new recommondations.

It is essential that dietary advice is consistent; are we all recommending wholemeal bread, potatoes in their jackets and polyunsaturated fats? The high carbohydrate diet demands more time than the conventional restricted carbohydrate diet and more attention has to be given to total energy intake. Printed diet sheets of 120 g, 150 g and 200 g carbohydrate diets are discouraged and should be replaced by a simple format giving the skeleton on which the individual diet can be based.

The nurse specialist in diabetes must have an understanding of nutrition and the principles that underly the diabetic diet, conversely the dietician must have an understanding of diabetes and current modes of therapy, particularly in relation to insulin administration and action. No one professional group cares for the person with diabetes but a team of professionals each contributing their own particular expertise and experience.

THE ROLE OF THE CHIROPODIST

Ischaemic or neuropathic complications affecting the foot are the single greatest cause of hospital admission for the diabetic. The pain and enforced immobility exacts a tremendous toll and the cost, financially, to the health service is not inconsiderable. Foot problems appear to have a social significance in as much as they most commonly afflict those in the lower income group, particularly the elderly living alone or with an equally elderly spouse. Are there any conclusions to be drawn from this observation? How do those in the higher social groups differ from the lower income groups in this context? First of all, from the point of view of hygiene they bathe more frequently, change their hose more often and possess more than one pair of shoes, and what is more their shoes are more likely to be made of leather. Those in the higher social classes may have a better understanding of the long-term effects of diabetes on nerves and blood vessels, and be more aware of the chiropody services available in the private sector and of the services available in the community. In this group, small lesions are identified early and treatment instituted before the condition worsens and requires more drastic intervention. There may be other more obscure differences including better nutrition and better self-esteem. The chiropodist has a two-fold function in the care of diabetic patients. Primarily, their function is to prevent foot problems by giving advice on self-care, for example—how often feet should be washed and the temperature of the water; care with drying feet, particularly between the toes; the application of a simple handcream to keep the skin soft and supple; treating moist skin between the toes with surgical spirit; how toe nails should or should not be cut and stressing that those with impaired vision, hard or painful nails or those suffering from arthritis should seek the aid of a state registered chiropodist. Advice about footwear is of paramount importance and the chiropodist is the most qualified person to do this.

Established neuropathy can deform the feet giving rise to the so-called claw-foot. Weight is unevenly distributed and concentrated onto the metatarsal heads, eventually leading to callous formation and corns on the toes. Corn plasters and paints are discouraged and skin parers are an anathema for the patient with sensory loss. Early referral to a chiropodist can do much to prevent further deterioration. Debridement of a foot ulcer and regular paring of the keratotic rim of the ulcer can assist with healing and special sponge-rubber insoles can help to redistribute the pressure away from the affected area. Ideally, there should be a close liaison between the chiropodist and the orthopaedic surgeon and between the chiropodist and the surgical shoemaker.

Many diabetic centres have a chiropodist as part of the clinic staff and referral of patients by the physicians is relatively easy. Regrettably, this is not always the case and delay in referral may affect morbidity and the success of the chiropody treatment. Consultation between the chiropodist, the patient and the physician may take place on a monthly basis until the chiropodist is satisfied with the progress of the patient. The chiropodist should ideally form part of the educational team and be involved much earlier in the teaching of foot-care.

The cost of not providing access to chiropody services may be great to the community but to the individual patient it may come to be measured in amputated digits or limbs.

WHICH TYPE OF CLINIC?

Introduction

Hospital clinics caring for diabetic patients were amongst the first specialised clinics established in hospitals. In recent years the idea that the care of the diabetic patient should be supervised by a hospital clinic has come under attack. Diabetes mellitus is a common disorder and this ensures a large clinical load in a hospital diabetic clinic. In turn this raises numerous problems. Patients may have to wait many hours to see the doctor and freqently complain that it is not possible to see the same doctor twice. The sheer numbers of diabetics attending the clinic may mean that the doctor has insufficient time to devote to difficult cases or to important features such as detecting diabetic retinopathy or examining patients' feet.

The alternative to hospital-based supervision of care is for care to be based in the community. In the U.K. a number of ways for organising this care have been described with quite major differences between them.

Mini-clinics in general practice

In the early 1970s mini-clinics were established in the Wolverhampton area as a combined operation between the local general practitioners and the hospital consultant. Within the participating clinics one or two general practitioners in a practice accepted that they would take a special interest in the care of the diabetic. In addition, the practice had to set aside one session per month for a diabetic clinic. At the outset patients were discharged from the hospital diabetic clinic if they were members of a participating practice. Perhaps reflecting a cautious approach initially, those discharged were mainly the older diabetics whose treatment consisted of diet or oral agents and only half of the patients in the participating practices who were on insulin therapy were discharged for care in the community.

As new diabetic patients were diagnosed all were initially seen in the hospital diabetic clinic, and it was generally agreed that this was a most useful feature. A first attendance at the hospital clinic allowed for a uniform approach to treatment in the area. In addition hospital records could be established and base-line recordings made which would be of great value in case of admission to hospital in the future. It also allowed the patient's contact with the clinic health visitor and the chiropodist. Following this initial consultation the general practitioner was entirely responsible for the continuing care of these patients. Only if the practitioner thought referral to hospital for consultation necessary did the patient reattend the hospital diabetic clinic.

Certain features reflecting the enthusiasm of the hospital specialist involved, contributed considerably to the success of these clinics. An annual visit by him to each of the mini-clinics was welcomed since it provided an opportunity for consultation and discussion of individual patients and diabetes in general. In addition his organisation of a monthly evening meeting attended by the general practitioners involved has helped considerably to maintain their enthusiasm.

It is held that this scheme provides advantages to both the general practitioner and his patients. Advantages to the practitioner of being responsible for his own diabetic patients enables an interest to be maintained in the disorder. Previously, removal of patients to a hospital clinic quite naturally led to a fading of interest. For the patients the advantages are that they are seen in more comfort with less waiting time in a more familiar environment than they encounter at hospital. In addition the same doctor is seen on each attendance.

All of the medical people involved in these mini-clinics feel that a better service is being provided than when the patients attended the hospital clinic.

The establishment and development of this scheme for mini-clinics has provided important guide-lines for the setting up of

Table 4.3 Essentials for the establishment of a mini-clinic

1. An interested practitioner in the group
2. An interested, involved practice nurse
3. Frequency of one clinic per month
4. System for regular review
5. Special record card
6. Liaison with the hospital

similar clinic arrangements. The pre-requisites for success are listed in Table 4.3. and the most important of these must be the involvement of an interested medical practitioner and an interested practice nurse. Then there must be a system whereby the patient finds it difficult to default from attending. Interestingly, it is emminently clear from the comparison of the patients attending the hospital compared with the patients

Name	NHS No.
Address	Hospital No.
	Age Date of Birth

Occupation

M. F.   M. S. W.

| Date | FAMILY HISTORY |

Evidence for Diagnosis

Year   Age

H. K. W.. lbs.

PRESENT WT. .... lbs.

HEIGHT .... ins.

STANDARD WT.............................. lbs.

Clinical State

RELATION OF PRESENT WT.
                    TO STANDARD WT.

.................................% ABOVE

Treatment Policy

.................................% BELOW

USUAL DIET

SUGAR   BREAD

CHO.

Figure 4.3a Record card of attendance at a diabetic clinic. The card serves as a liaison card between hospital and mini-clinic. First attendance.

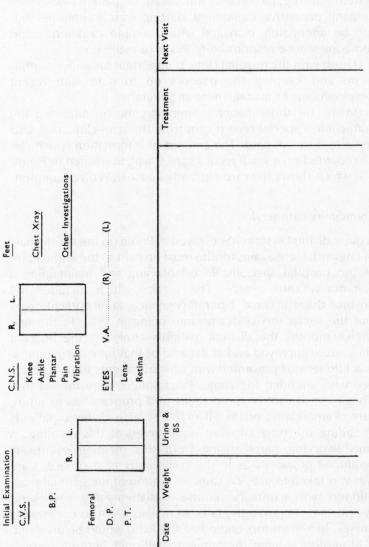

Initial Examination

C.V.S.

B.P.

Femoral

D.P.

P.T.

R. L.

C.N.S.

Knee
Ankle
Plantar
Pain
Vibration

EYES

V.A. (R) .... (L)

Lens

Retina

Feet

R. L.

Chest Xray

Other Investigations

Date	Weight	Urine & BS		Treatment	Next Visit

Figure 4.3b Follow-up.

attending the general practitioner that defaulters are more frequent in the first group. It must be stressed that devising a system for regular review and recall of patients does not demand expensive equipment starting with a computer but can be adequately managed with a simple card index and someone whose responsibility this is to maintain.

Liaison with the hospital clinic is important for policy, enthusiasm and keeping the patients up to date with recent developments in management and therapy.

Finally, for those patients attending the hospital and the mini-clinic a special record card from the mini-clinic may also serve as a liaison card. The amount of information which can be recorded on a small record card is well illustrated in Figure 4.3. which shows the card currently in use in Wolverhampton.

Community care service

A quite distinct system has evolved in Poole on the south coast of England. Here again, tribute must be paid to the enthusiasm of the hospital specialist in establishing and maintaining a community care service. The service which includes the hospital diabetic clinic, laboratory service, family practitioners and the social services came into being in 1970. In the first twelve months the diabetic patients attending the hospital clinic were surveyed and at the end of that time each general practitioner was presented with a list of patients from his practice who attended the clinic. Practitioners were invited to a discussion of care of the diabetic and proposals as to future care. Remarkably, nearly all practices with diabetic patients attending the hospital were represented at this meeting. A small working party arising from this meeting eventually produced proposals as to the community care service. Care was was taken to provide some education of the general practitioners with a refresher course in diabetes and a weekend symposium. Importantly, talks were also given to community nurses, health visitors and other staff who would be involved.

In another system the family practitioner became responsible for the detection of new diabetics and their referral to the hospital clinic for assessment and registration. He also undertook follow-up of selected known diabetics including assessing their metabolic control and detection of complications.

Follow-up and care in the home by health visitors and community nurses fell within the province of the general practitioner to arrange; however, chiropody or dietetic advice remained within the orbit of the hospital diabetic clinic.

The majority of patients being cared for in this way are non-insulin-dependent diabetics. Typically they are free from diabetic complications as are the few insulin-requiring diabetic patients managed in this manner.

The care of many patients in the community allows the hospital diabetic clinic a change of direction. It has been stressed that the workload of the diabetic clinic at the hospital has not decreased but considerably more time is now spent on detecting complications of diabetes, particularly diabetic retinopathy and neuropathy. The system has been introduced whereby the patients remain under the supervision of the general practitioner but may be recalled at given time intervals for screening for complications.

Similar advantages for patients have been recorded from this clinic arrangement. Questionnaires sent out to patients indicate a marked preference for having their own doctor look after them. This is true even in those who were initially reluctant to leave the hospital diabetic clinic. Family practitioners have also enjoyed increasing their expertise in treating diabetes. Benefits to the hospital diabetic clinic must be that more time can be given to the detection of diabetic complications.

What is missing from both the Wolverhampton and the Poole systems is an assessment of the standard of diabetic control and the effect upon this of the different schemes. It would seem extremely unlikely that the management of diabetic patients in the community has resulted in any deterioration in diabetic control and indeed it is likely that an overall improvement in care has occurred.

The peripatetic clinic

The two schemes described above are the ones of which most experience has been gained. Several other groups or practices have attempted their own variations of community diabetic clinics and one of the recently introduced larger schemes is the peripatetic clinic. In the peripatetic clinic the hospital team of medical, nursing and biochemistry staff are taken out into the community to the practices. This allows small clinics to reduce travel and waiting time for patients and helps to establish a close liaison with primary health care workers. The scheme is particularly suited to rural areas with poor public transport facilities.

Alternatives

Many attempts have been made to discharge the so called 'mild' diabetic patient to the care of their general practitioners. These have met with varying degrees of success. One of the major problems lies in identifying those patients who have mild diabetes. In one of the many apposite quotations of Dr Arnold Bloom he points out that what is generally termed mild diabetes is similar to mild cigarettes in that they can both severely damage your health! One of the major advantages of the schemes described above arises from the enthusiasm of the supervisory hospital specialist. Their prompting, cajoling, and at times badgering, ensures a uniform standard of care throughout the practices in their area. This is not always the case as is revealed by an audit of standards of diabetic care carried out in 1976 in one general practice. This showed that 52 per cent of known diabetics were totally unsupervised either by the hospital or general practitioner, and 47 per cent of those with complications were not seen regularly.

Rather more disturbingly and somewhat of an antidote to the enthusiasm with which community care schemes are greeted, is the experience recorded in Cardiff. Here a study was commenced involving randomised discharge of diabetics to general practitioners. Prior to the onset of the study the local general practitioners and the hospital had a number of meetings discussing the aims of diabetic care in general practice. Analysis of their results shows that only 4 per cent of diabetic patients discharged to the care of the general practitioner had a blood glucose measurement done each year. Furthermore, this 4 per cent attended a practice of one of the general practitioners who worked in the hospital diabetic clinic. Only 19 per cent of the patients were being seen by their general practitioners on a regular basis with a minimum visit of once per year. For the remainder of patients discharged from the hospital there was no semblance of any form of follow-up. The conclusions of this study are clear. Diabetic patients can only be discharged to the care of the general practitioner if the practice are prepared to make a special effort towards regular review, eye examination, and blood glucose measurement. Clearly practices that are prepared to make these special arrangements tend to have an interest in the care of the diabetic.

What then can we say in conclusion of the forms of community care for the diabetic patient which have been attempted. We can say that the system works in areas where general practitioners are interested and motivated by a desire to care for their own patients within the community. Where general practitioners are not of this mind, community care is patchy and may at times be non-existent. Wholesale discharge of patients from the hospital diabetic clinic, therefore, is not a feasible proposition unless in particular areas. Other than this, limited discharge of patients will depend upon the hospital specialist's knowledge of the general practitioners in his area. Such knowledge is easier to obtain in smaller towns or cities than in the large cities such as London and Birmingham.

In most large clinics a compromise has been reached whereby the majority of patients have been retained and certain patients discharged to selected general practitioners.

The answer to the question 'do we need large hospital-based diabetic clinics?' must be 'yes!'. In these clinics the medical, nursing and dietetic staff benefit from their exposure to all manifestations of the disease. The hospital becomes the centre of expertise and certain groups of patients will always require specialist care. Pregnant women, children, adolescents, many insulin-dependent diabetics and those classified as 'brittle' as well as those requiring treatment for complications all fall into this category. There can be little doubt that centralisation of care is of benefit to pregnant diabetics. The marked reduction in mortality of the infants from insulin-dependent diabetic mothers has been largely brought about by the joint hospital-based clinics run by physicians and obstetricians. In addition, large hospital clinics will always be necessary for the development of screening techniques and research into new treatments.

The size and type of the clinic depends to a large extent on population density and geographical location. To discharge patients to the care of general practitioners, thus allowing more time for screening, for example for diabetic retinopathy, is desirable but only feasible where there are adequate resources and interest in the community.

ORGANISATION OF DIABETIC CARE

B. IN-PATIENT CARE

Introduction

Having dealt in the previous sections with the organisation of care for the diabetic patient as an out-patient, we can now turn to the organisation of in-patient care. Our first considerations must be the reasons for which diabetic patients are admitted to hospital. These can be grouped under three headings as in Table 4.4. There will be little argument about the first two reasons in the table. Acute emergencies which necessitate hospital admission include diabetic ketoacidosis and other hyperglycaemic comas. At other times it may be necessary to admit patients with acute hypoglycaemic episodes. Secondly, diabetic patients may be admitted because of the complications of diabetes which necessitate specific treatments. The final broad reason for admission of diabetic patients is for stabilisation and education. The fact that this is third on our list does not imply that it is less important than the two preceding reasons. It is more contentious, however, as will be seen when it is discussed later in this section.

Table 4.4 Reasons for admitting diabetic patients to hospital

1. Diabetic emergencies
2. Assessment and treatment of the patient with complications of diabetes
3. Education and stabilisation of the diabetic patient

Diabetic emergencies

Hypoglycaemia

The vast majority of diabetic patients cope with hypoglycaemia themselves or with the help of relatives or friends without recourse to medical assistance. The recognition of hypoglycaemic episodes and their early treatment are an essential part of education programmes for newly diagnosed diabetic patients and it is often surprising how patients who have had diabetes for some years are still unsure about how they should deal with hypoglycaemic episodes. Coma resulting from hypoglycaemia demands urgent treatment. Medical assistance is usually necessary if an intravenous injection of 50 per cent dextrose is to be used to rouse the patient. The difficulties and dangers of an intravenous injection of this viscous fluid should not be underestimated in a patient who may be confused or aggressive. It is perhaps for this reason, as well as for the reason that medical assistance may be difficult to obtain or delayed, that more and more relatives of patients are being taught in the use of glucagon injections. Glucagon can be given by subcutaneous injection, intramuscular injection, or intravenous injection and there is little reason therefore why a nurse should not accept responsibility for treating a hypoglycaemic coma. In this way, the community nurse may make unnecessary a visit to the local hospital Casualty Department. Should the patient reach a Casualty Department, the hypoglycaemic coma must firstly be recognised and secondly be treated. In the majority of cases this presents few problems and most hospital Casualty Departments are familiar with some regular attenders. The diagnosis should always be suspected when casualty staff receive any hint that the patient may be a diabetic. This may simply include the fact that the patient is carrying an out-patient diabetic card or has on their person dextrosol or similar substance. It is important for staff to realise that hypoglycaemic coma may present in an unusual way, for example as a cerebrovascular accident. With the rapid measurement of blood glucose by reagent stix there is no reason why every diabetic entering a Casualty Department should not have their blood glucose measured. It is perhaps safer to make this general rule than to list the many ways in which hypo-glycaemia may present.

With an intravenous injection of 50 per cent glucose most patients regain consciousness within a few minutes. Delayed response may indicate transitory changes in the brain. Many patients attending the Casualty Department with hypogly-caemic coma do not need hospital admission. Consciousness is restored speedily and further hypoglycaemic episodes are prevented by ensuring that the patients receive a meal. It must be remembered that treating a hypoglycaemic episode by glucose alone may be inadequate. The glucose may be rapidly metabolised, and it is necessary to ensure maintenance of blood glucose concentration by providing carbohydrate in a form which is absorbed over a longer period of time. Poor recovery from a hypoglycaemic coma is a reason for hospital admission. In similar manner, a prolonged severe hypogly-caemic episode is a reason for admission to hospital. What constitutes a prolonged or severe hypoglycaemic episode may vary from patient to patient. It is clear that an elderly patient experiencing a hypoglycaemic episode who lives alone may need hospital admission, while a similar episode in a younger person may not prompt this decision. Junior medical staff in Casualty often pay insufficient attention to this point. The prompt recovery and discharge from the Casualty Department of a young patient establishes a pattern which the young doctor expects will extend to the older patient. It is unsatis-factory to keep elderly patients lying on a Casualty trolley for most of the day waiting for full recovery from a hypoglycaemic episode.

Recognition and treatment is often all that is attempted by the staff of the Casualty Department. It should not be forgotten, however, that the hypoglycaemic episode was caused by some factor which attempts should be made to identify. A change in insulin dosage or diet may be necessary, and a patient should not be left to continue with the same dose of insulin without first considering all the contributory factors. It may be necessary to ask if there has been a change of insulin syringe or strength of insulin. Has there been a recent change in the type of insulin, from beef to pork or human insulin? This may have been a therapeutic change made by the general prac-titioner or in the clinic but we must also remember that occasionally mistakes are made in dispensing insulin and in view of the number of preparations currently on the market this is hardly surprising. Temporary changes in insulin requirement may come about during the 'honeymoon period' when the recovery of endogenous insulin secretion follows diagnosis. At times during the menstrual cycle many women experience transitory changes in their insulin requirement. This is well worth being identified by the nurse or doctor if the patient has not observed the relationship herself. Missed or delayed meals are a common cause of hypoglycaemic episodes—and there are many reasons for these. A child may have found a new adventure which is irresistable, an adolescent or young adult may have been to a party the night before and consumed considerable amounts of alcohol, while with the elderly a late arrival of the meals-on-wheels service may be sufficient for hypoglycaemia to occur. All of the reasons for the hypoglcaemic episode are worthy of identification. Further education of the patient with regard to regularity of meals or consumption of alcohol may be of benefit, while third parties responsible for providing meals, such as meals-on-wheels or school dinners, may be reminded of the importance of timing. Finally, we should probably ask that all patients who experience a hypoglycaemic episode in the absence of an obvious precipitating factor should draw up their insulin and show the nurse the dose that is being administered. Only in this way will the patient who may be visually handicapped and who may simply be guessing the amount of insulin be brought to light. We must not forget that to many people admitting that they have difficulty with their own injection may mean a loss of independence. Patients may not be aware of aids for the visually handicapped but are all too well aware that a number of people need injections to be given daily by a district nurse. They feel that their independence will be lost in this way and it is not surprising that they are loath to demonstrate their frailties.

Hyperglycaemic emergencies

Pathogenesis and treatment of diabetic ketoacidosis and hyperosmolar non-ketotic coma have been discussed elsewhere in this volume (Ch. 6). Since hyperglycaemic emergencies are life-threatening, hospital admission is imperative and while not discussing here the specific aspects of treatment, we should consider how the management of these emergencies should be organised. Two arguments surface at this stage. On one side of the argument are people who believe that treatment should be carried out in an intensive care unit or high-dependency ward by a skilled and experienced team of doctors, nurses, and clinical biochemistry staff. The opposing view is that by managing acute emergencies in this way the general pool of knowledge amongst medical and nursing staff is depleted. This view would argue that the hyperglycaemic emergencies should be treated by whichever medical firm they happen to be admitted under and on whichever medical ward this firm admits its patients. There can be little doubt, however, that the mortality from diabetic ketoacidosis is lower when patients are managed in the first of these two ways. On the face of it, it would appear that enhancing the general level of knowledge of medical and nursing staff should take second place to the acute interests of the patient. This argument is not as solid as it first appears. If we leave the treatment of acute diabetic emergencies to specialist staff, we must remember that the majority of doctors and nurses do not work in specialised units. Neither do the majority of patients live within easy reach of a specialised unit. It is, therefore, in the longer term interests of diabetic patients that as many medical and nursing staff as possible be exposed to all aspects of the disease and especially that they should have sufficient knowledge to appreciate the seriousness of certain aspects of the condition. This debate currently runs through the whole of medicine. Gastroenterologists may feel that gastrointestinal haemorrhage is best dealt with in a specialist unit; respiratory physicians may feel that respiratory failure should be dealt with in their specialist unit; the argument cannot be resolved and is a consequence of super-specialisation which has occurred in the teaching hospitals.

Either method of managing the acute emergency should make provision for specialist advice. This may be in the acute phase of rehydration and insulin therapy and should certainly be in the phase following restoration of metabolic normality. A proportion of the diabetic patients presenting with ketoacidosis do so as newly diagnosed diabetic patients. This may indicate that earlier symptoms and signs of diabetes may have been missed or misinterpreted. Such patients and their families will require a full educational programme and psychological support to meet the stress of an acute illness followed by the realisation that the patient has a chronic disease requiring life-long treatment. Here, the specialist nurse or a nurse with an interest in diabetes can play a major part.

Following the initial treatment of the acute episode the established diabetic patient will require restabilising and most probably re-educating. Identification of the precipitating factor for diabetic ketoacidosis is important. A considerable proportion present without obvious precipitating cause and in these patients the hours preceding admission should be carefully gone over. Emphasis should be placed on the appropriate time for the patient to seek medical assistance. Judicious use of blood tests or of urine tests for glucose and ketones, combined with advice on alterations in insulin therapy, may be invaluable in saving this patient from future episodes of this life-threatening disorder.

Repeated admissions with diabetic ketoacidosis may signal 'brittle' diabetes. Every series of patients with diabetic ketoacidosis, which is reported in the literature, of any appreciable number has one or two patients who account for more than their fair share of episodes of diabetic ketoacidosis in the series. Brittle diabetes (Ch. 6.) may have a physiological basis but it may also intimate underlying social or emotional problems. The doctor, enjoying the manipulation of intravenous fluid and the dose of insulin, may not have the same enthusiasm in tackling the social or emotional problems of his patient. Indeed, when faced with this situation the doctor may be an inappropriate confidante who merely wishes to get on with the rest of the ward round. The indispensibility of an interested nurse in this situation is well illustrated in the following two case histories from our own clinic.

Anne is a 19-year-old insulin-dependent diabetic patient who was diagnosed at the age of 5 years. She went through a phase of numerous admissions in diabetic ketoacidosis for which no definite precipitating cause could be found. On each occasion that she was admitted to the hospital she was escorted by her parents and her fiancé. It would have been easy to decide that this situation would continue as long as Anne had either the same mother or the same boyfriend. An experienced Ward Sister, however, decided to tackle it head on. She attempted to reconstruct the twenty-four hours prior to the admission in diabetic ketoacidosis. There was always one thing in common—a serious row between mother and daughter. At this point we could safely blame the daughter for her response to a family argument. Further questioning, however, revealed that the mother was suffering from menopausal depression and was almost impossible to live with. It is perhaps best that we fail to recall whether specific advice was given. However, for the few remaining months before her marriage, Anne decided to live with an aunt. No further episodes of diabetic ketoacidosis occurred either during this time or since her marriage. She has had two normal pregnancies and both during these and after these she managed her diabetes in an exemplary way.

Rosie, a 17-year-old insulin-dependent diabetic patient had numerous admissions in diabetic ketoacidosis. Again, no apparent cause could be found. The episodes had started, however, following the move of Rosie's parents from city-centre housing to an overspill area. Rosie had decided not to leave her friends but to live with an unmarried sister and her baby in a council flat. Following this, she experienced several episodes of diabetic ketoacidosis and was usually profoundly acidotic on admission. On each occasion the medical aspect of treatment was straightforward. The ultimate question, however, was how were these episodes to be prevented before Rosie did herself harm. Her parents were approached and they urged her to return to the family home. She declined this, but such was the concern that the health visitor and medical social worker were asked to visit Rosie in her flat. They eventually discovered that once the social security money had been spent on clothes, cosmetics, a huge dog, and the current boyfriend, there was little money left by the end of the week for food. Given this situation, and rather than risk hypoglycaemic episodes, Rosie discontinued her insulin. Shortly after this she would need admitting for ketoacidosis.

The situation was resolved by the amount of persuasion and pressure brought to bear on Rosie in that she eventually returned to the parental home.

Patients with complications of diabetes

In Chapter 2 we discussed the relationship of diabetic control to the development of complications. The evidence suggests that improved metabolic control may be advantageous for those patients with evidence of early complications, e.g. background retinopathy. Improved blood glucose control may retard the progression of the retinopathy and prepare the patient for possible ophthalmic intervention. Whether such patients are admitted to hospital in order to achieve improved control of blood glucose is arguable. The very nature of life spent in hospital with controlled meals and limited exercise makes it remote from the normal daily life of many patients. Many would argue that in these circumstances attempts to improve diabetic control should be made with the patient in their normal environment. This is a similar argument to that which will be discussed later in this section about whether newly diagnosed insulin-dependent diabetic patients should be admitted.

At certain times disability due to the complications of diabetes may necessitate hospital admission. Foot problems are probably the greatest cause for admission to hospital for the diabetic patient although other consequences of large and small vessel disease and damage to nerves do at times result in in-patient care.

Renal disease

Patients with renal damage due to diabetes may be admitted either because of the chronic renal failure or because of the effect of this upon diabetic control. Renal damage can seriously affect the management of diabetes. Insulin is excreted by the kidney and a damaged kidney will therefore excrete less efficiently, thus increasing the half-life of insulin in the circulation. In chronic renal failure, anorexia or nausea and vomiting may be a problem and the patient's dietary intake may decrease because of this. Gluconeogenesis in the kidney makes a small contribution to maintaining blood glucose concentration; however, under certain circumstances the importance of this pathway is increased. It is likely that there is some impairment if the kidney is damaged. All of these contribute to a reduction in insulin requirement with the establishment and development of chronic renal failure. Simultaneously, other changes make manipulation of insulin dose difficult. Changes in the renal threshold for glucose suggest that such patients should not rely on urine testing as a guide to control but should use blood glucose monitoring. Many patients are puzzled by the changes in their insulin requirements and should be given a careful explanation.

Regular assessment of a patient with chronic renal failure due to diabetic nephropathy should be an important part of the management of the condition. In recent years the resistance to offering renal dialysis or transplantation to patients with diabetes has decreased. This does not mean that all our diabetic patients with chronic renal failure should be offered one of these two alternatives. It seems incumbent upon us to use this service responsibly. If we are to do this then we must know our patients well, know their capabilities and their limitations. We should also be careful about talking of the possibility of renal transplantation if this is not likely to materialise either because of inadequate resources or because ultimately the patient is felt to be unsuitable for such a procedure. Full assessment, therefore, based on knowledge of the patient and of the progression of the patient's disease is necessary to make a responsible decision.

In addition, certain features of the disorder should be identified and treated long before the question of dialysis or transplantation occurs. In particular the control of hypertension secondary to the renal damage clearly delays the progression of further renal damage. Furthermore, infections should be treated early and enthusiastically before they result in further tissue damage. More and more diabetic patients, however, with end stage diabetic renal failure are being referred for dialysis. In many centres this takes the form of continuous ambulatory peritoneal dialysis. Peritoneal dialysis was first used as early as 1923 but the continuous ambulatory variety of this was introduced as recently as 1975. As the name implies, the process is continuous and yet allows the patient freedom of movement while the dialysis is proceeding. A permanent catheter is implanted in the abdominal wall with one end resting in the peritoneal cavity and the other end fitted with an adaptor to accept the dialysing administration set. Dialysing fluid is infused from a plastic container similar to plastic intravenous infusion bags. The exchange of fluids takes approximately 30 minutes and in between the exchanges the patient is free to carry out normal activities. Peritonitis is a serious hazard but this has been reduced by an improvement in the technique and in the apparatus. Again, it should be stressed that careful selection of patients is important. The element of self-care involved means that the success or failure of this treatment depends on the patient's motivation as well as upon sound nursing and medical back-up services.

For the diabetic patient on chronic ambulatory peritoneal dialysis insulin is usually added to the dialysing fluid. The amount of insulin added is determined by the concentration of glucose in the dialysing fluid and may vary from as little as 4 units to as much as 30 units per litre bag four times daily. Good diabetic control can be achieved in this manner and the procedure also has the advantages of ease of administration, and insulin absorption via the protal vein. A number of studies have shown that with the use of home blood glucose monitoring, patients or their spouses can learn to adjust insulin dosage to produce good diabetic control.

For some years, patients with renal failure due to diabetic nephropathy were considered unsuitable for renal transplantation. Since it was also felt that they fared worse than non-diabetic patients with chronic renal failure on peritoneal or haemodialysis the serious nature of chronic renal failure due to chronic diabetic nephropathy was obvious. More recently dialysis, particularly continuous ambulatory peritoneal dialysis, has been used with good effect in patients with diabetic nephropathy. It is not clear, however, whether this provides a long-term solution to chronic renal failure due to diabetes. Indeed, it seems likely that diabetic patients with their susceptibility to infection may experience a higher incidence of peritoneal infections. It is necessary, therefore, to continue to consider renal transplantation in the diabetic. Kidney transplants are well known to occur by the lay public and it is therefore not surprising to hear relatives of patients asking about the possibility of a transplant.

The decision to offer a diabetic patient a renal transplant should be made jointly by the diabetologist, nephrologist, and the transplant surgeon. These are not the people who are likely to be asked by relatives about a transplant. It is therefore important that the nurse should appreciate the local policy on renal transplantation for diabetics. There remain specific factors which can be disadvantageous for transplantation in the diabetic patient. Atheroma of blood vessels can add to the difficulties of anastomoses and transplant patients, *per se*, have an increased thrombotic tendency. In addition the emotional and metabolic stress imposed by the major surgery together with immuno-suppressant therapy may dramatically worsen diabetic control. The major drugs responsible for this are the steroid family. It is therefore of considerable interest to the diabetic patient to hear of the development of non-steroidal immunosuppressive therapy such as Cyclosporin A.

If your patient does get as far as a renal transplantation diabetes can be managed during the procedure using an intra-venous infusion pump or intravenous insulin via a drip set. Post-operatively it is easy to give small amounts of insulin frequently and it is not unusual to find patients being given 2 to 4 units insulin hourly by either the intramuscular or subcu-taneous injection route, depending upon blood glucose concentration. Frequent and regular blood glucose estima-tions are essential during the initial post-operative period. As an interesting aside it has been noted that tuberculosis may come to light in the post-operative period presumably unmasked by immunosuppressant therapy. In some centres it has become policy to prescribe anti-tubercular therapy prophylactically.

The success rate for renal transplantation is dependent upon the source of the donor organ, suppression of rejection, and the avoidance of disease in the new kidney. An example of the importance of these factors is that renal transplantation between identical twins leads to a 90 per cent, ten year survival both for the kidney and for the patient, whereas only 50 per cent of cadaver kidneys are functioning after one year, and 30 per cent of patients who receive a kidney from a cadaver die within one year. Despite these somewhat depressing figures, the advantages of a successful transplant are paramount. For the diabetic patient it is the difference between an early death and survival, between the inconvenience of long-term dialysis and freedom, between despair and well-being. Not every patient will be suitable, however, and limited resources and kidney shortage will probably tend to keep diabetic patients low on the list of priorities at least in the immediate future.

One foot-note should be added. The question often arises as to whether complications of diabetes occur in the trans-planted kidney. We should consider the success if the patient survives long enough for this to happen. Small vessel disease does indeed occur in the transplanted kidney but only after five to ten years.

Neuropathic complications

Three aspects of nerve disease due to diabetes warrant admission from time to time.

Firstly, certain types of diabetic neuropathy may be painful. This is particularly true of diabetic amyotrophy which often affects middle-aged or elderly patients. The pain of this condition may be excruciating, a fact which is not always appreciated by general practitioners. Sadly, it is a general rule that these patients receive inadequate analgesia. Physicians are reluctant to prescribe opiate drugs in an apparently chronic condition. This often means that by the time the patient has been referred back to the diabetic clinic, he or she may be exhausted due to lack of sleep and often close to despair because of pain. It is at this time that admission to hospital may be beneficial in that it provides time to assess the extent of the neuropathy and exclude other conditions if necessary, to control the pain, and to assess and improve diabetic control. Considerable and often dramatic relief can be achieved by improving blood glucose levels. This may necessitate transferring patients from oral hypoglycaemic agents to insulin, or insulin-dependent patients from once or twice daily insulin to more frequent injections. Considerable success has been achieved in some centres by using continuous subcutaneous infusions of insulin in selected patients. While this medical manipulation is in progress there is a significant role for the nursing staff. The opportunity should be grasped with both hands to reinforce the importance of foot care. The dangers of trauma cannot be overemphasised whether due to ill-fitting shoes, exposure to heat or cold, or the hazards of amateur chiropody.

In this condition tight diabetic control is aimed at. This is similar to the degree of control which is demanded in a pregnant diabetic patient. In order to achieve this degree of control a number of variables must be reduced to the minimum. This emphasises the importance of checks being made on the patient's injection technique, injection sites, equipment, and insulin. Effects of varying the technique or the site of injections should be explained carefully to the patient.

The second type of painful motor neuropathy may occur in young people and often in those whose adolescent career was chequered by numerous admisssions for diabetic ketoacidosis. It is likely that this painful disorder is due to disease of many nerves and indeed the pains may be in the legs and feet or in the arms and hands. Again the treatment of choice is to improve diabetic control and to provide adequate analgesia. In addition it may be necessary at times to splint painful limbs or parts of limbs. The nurse should be aware that this is a hazardous practice and should only be combined with intelligent physiotherapy advice. The injudicious splinting of limbs may accentuate the muscle wasting due to pain-induced lack of use.

Autonomic neuropathy is amongst the most disabling of complications of diabetes. The signs and symptoms are so diverse that many patients thus afflicted will require hospital treatment at some stage. The problems are recurrent and the treatment merely palliative. The full range of problems due to autonomic neuropathy is covered in Chapter 3. There is little evidence that an improvement in control of blood glucose concentration will improve autonomic neuropathy. Nevertheless, it may retard the progress of the disorder and to many physicians would be a logical aim of treatment. Here a special problem arises. One of the features of longstanding autonomic neuropathy is a loss of hypoglycaemic awareness. This may devastate a diabetic patient's life and the extent of mortality from such a problem has not been defined but may well be significant. The uncertainty induced in a patient by loss of warning of hypoglycaemic attacks is usually underestimated by the physician. Patients who have to face this problem need considerable support and education. Hypoglycaemic attacks should be recalled by the patient and nurse in an attempt to find one small but persistent warning of impending hypoglycaemia. If this proves impossible then the customary important advice on avoidance of hypos should be reiterated until it is apparent that the patient has a good grasp of it. Home blood glucose monitoring may be of considerable benefit and the use of glucagon by a spouse or relative to rapidly curtail an attack should not be neglected. A further problem in this area is that the same patient may experience postural hypotension. This can be a distressing phenomenon confining the patient to a wheelchair simply because standing upright results in a loss of consciousness. In less extreme circumstances the patient may simply feel light-headed when standing or sitting-up and the nature of this should be clearly explained. It is not uncommon to find patients or their relatives confusing the symptoms of postural hypotension with those previously recognised for hypoglycaemia. To treat the latter when the symptoms originate from the former may result in astronomic elevation of blood glucose levels.

Some years ago the doctors at King's College Hospital in London drew attention to unexplained cardiorespiratory arrests occurring in diabetic patients during anaesthesia. It is felt that autonomic neuropathy contributes considerably to this event. We should be aware of this problem and it would be sensible if all our longstanding insulin-dependent diabetic patients were assessed for autonomic neuropathy before undergoing general anaesthesia. A similar programme might be suggested for non-insulin-dependent diabetic patients who have any suggestion of autonomic neuropathy. Most diabetic patients undergoing surgery do so successfully and we should not feel that this complication should preclude necessary surgical treatment. The awareness that such patients form a high-risk group, however, should indicate that a more careful assessment pre-operatively and careful monitoring during surgery should be adopted.

Other problems with autonomic neuropathy may be equally disabling. It can only be reiterated that specific treatment of features of autonomic neuropathy is extremely non-specific and has generally poor results. As is often the case in medicine when such a situation exists, someone has to keep explaining to the patient why nothing is being done or why nothing is being achieved by the various treatments which are being tried. To explain this fully takes time and a sympathetic approach. It is clearly impossible for it to be done on a routine ward round by the medical team. Such miserable attempts are likely only to confuse the patient further and necessitate that the nurse spend considerable time with the patient following the conclusion of the round.

Complications due to large vessel disease—macroangiopathy

Myocardial infarction occurring in a diabetic patient presents special problems over and above those associated with the management of the infarction in non-diabetic patients. The recognition that the patient has sustained a myocardial infarction may be difficult due to the more frequent incidence of so-called 'silent' myocardial infarctions—that is pain free. Shock and congestive cardiac failure appear to occur more commonly in the diabetic patient than in the non-diabetic patient following myocardial infarction. All of these complications when occurring in a diabetic patient are dealt with in the same manner as in a non-diabetic patient. What is unique to the diabetic is the effect of the stress response. The biochemical nature of the stress response includes secretion of the hormones glucagon, cortisol, and particularly following myocardial infarction catecholamines. All these have effects which oppose those of insulin. This could be stated in an alternative way by saying that following a myocardial infarction a non-diabetic subject needs to secrete more insulin to overcome the effects of the stress hormones. In this way the biochemical stress response in non-diabetic subjects is limited, although it is not uncommon to find these patients showing moderate degrees of glycosuria. That they do not become frankly diabetic is because of their ability to increase insulin secretion. The majority of diabetic patients do not have this option. Thus in all diabetic patients, but particularly insulin-dependent diabetic patients, the biochemical stress response may be most marked with blood glucose rising to more than 20 mmol/l and ketones appearing in the serum and urine.

In order to counteract this effect of catabolic hormones, patients on diet or diet plus oral hypoglycaemic agents may need to be transferred to insulin therapy in the acute phase following a myocardial infarction. Insulin-dependent diabetic patients who sustain a myocardial infarction present major problems in the control of their blood glucose concentration.

In the acute stages of a myocardial infarction diabetic patients fare worse than non-diabetic patients—a point which should be borne in mind by the nurse when talking to relatives. Furthermore the outcome appears to be related to the blood glucose concentration at presentation. This is a correlation and we must be wary about drawing major conclusions from it. One interpretation would be that the higher your blood glucose concentration at presentation, i.e. the worse your diabetic control, the greater your chances of mishap in the acute phase following myocardial infarction. In general this correlation has been interpreted in this way. There is an alternative explanation, however, and that is that the greater your myocardial infarction the greater the stress response associated with it and the higher the blood glucose concentration will be pushed by the catabolic hormones. It is not clear which of these two explanations is likely to be correct. For this and a number of reasons, however, most physicians would argue that good control of blood glucose concentration is extremely important immediately following a myocardial infarction. The question then is, how do we achieve good control of blood glucose concentration?

As for the management of diabetes during surgery or labour in the diabetic woman, numerous regimens have been devised for controlling diabetes after myocardial infarction. A majority of these consist of giving small amounts of quick-acting insulin four to six hourly. The next dose of insulin is adjusted on the basis of the previous urine or blood tests. Even with careful supervision of such a regimen, however, blood glucose concentration may swing wildly. We recently introduced an insulin infusion regimen to our coronary care unit in an attempt to improve the management of diabetes after myocardial infarction. A Braun pump and 50 ml syringe are used and 16 units of quick-acting insulin (Actrapid or Velosulin) are added to 45 ml of 0.9 per cent saline (154 mmol/l). There has been considerable debate about adsorption of insulin to plastic syringes and tubing and to prevent this sticking of insulin to the surfaces we add 1 vial (2.5 ml) of human albumin to this solution. Our total volume, therefore, is 48 ml and we then give 1 unit or 2 units or 4 units per hour according to the blood glucose concentration. The full protocol is indicated in Table 4.5. An example of the change in blood glucose during insulin infusion according to the protocol is shown in Figure 4.4 when the patient was a 45-year-old man with insulin-dependent diabetes for 18 years. It is difficult to show that our diabetic patients are any better controlled after their myocardial infarction using this regimen than using our previous system

Table 4.5 Protocol for insulin infusion following myocardial infarction. Rapid-acting insulin (16 u) is diluted with 45 ml of 0.9 per cent saline (154 mmol/l). The flow and hence insulin concentration infused is indicated for a range of blood glucose measurement.

Clucose	Insulin	Flow
0–8 mmol/l	1 unit/hour	3 ml/hour
8–12 mmol/l	2 units/hour	6 ml/hour
12–24 mmol/l	4 units/hour	12 ml/hour

of short-acting insulin frequently. We tend to think that they are, but one of the clear advantages that emerges from this regimen is the preference which the nursing staff on the coronary care unit have for it. They find that the management of diabetes following myocardial infarction using this protocol is simple and effective. With the aid of reagent stix, blood glucose concentration can be checked hourly or less frequently depending upon changes which are occuring in the concentration. It is surprising to some doctors that they can be virtually dispensed with when clear simple instructions like these are followed. Only on occasions when blood glucose concentration at presentation exceeds 24 mmol/l is specific advice sought by the nurses. Even then they are normally able to tell the house officer that last time this occurred an infusion of 6 units or 8 units per hour was given. We have been delighted with the response of the nurses to this regimen and

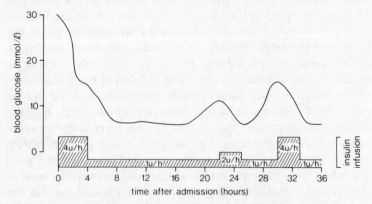

Figure 4.4 Changes in blood glucose concentration during insulin infusion in a 45-year-old insulin-dependent diabetic following myocardial infarction.

feel that it is easily within the compass of most coronary care units. We should add that often many fruitless hours are spent arguing about which insulin regimen for managing myocardial infarction or surgery or labour is preferable. There is no doubt that the regimen which is preferable is the one which in your hospital is the safest and most reliable.

Because the regimen has proved so straightforward we have tended to employ it for 48 to 72 hours post-infarction in those whose diabetes is difficult to control. They are then transferred back to subcutaneous therapy in the normal way.

Admission to hospital for education

We must return now to the question posed earlier in this chapter—whether the newly-diagnosed diabetic patient should be admitted to hospital for initial stabilisation and education. Similar discussion applies to whether patients should be admitted for restabilisation of their diabetes and re-education. It must be said that this is a contentious point. Clearly the decision is made for you if the patient presents in diabetic ketoacidosis or if your newly-diagnosed diabetic patient presents with complications of diabetes such as gangrene. The debate therefore revolves around the younger, newly-diagnosed insulin-dependent diabetic patient with signs and symptoms of diabetes, hyperglycaemia and probably ketonuria, but not to the extent which necessitates rehydration with intravenous fluids. Should such patients receive initial education and stabilisation of their diabetes in hospital or at home?

Admission to hospital

It is unfortunate, but a fact of life, that many of these newly diagnosed insulin-dependent diabetic patients often have to be admitted to large medical wards with acutely ill, dying or confused patients. If within the hospital there is no alternative, every endeavour should be made to allow the patient to be up and dressed during the daytime, to visit local shops, and to have weekend leave. We must recall that the vast majority of these patients do not feel particularly ill on admission and certainly feel remarkably fit and well after the first 24–36 hours of insulin therapy. Few hospitals are fortunate to have a small ward specifically designated to the care of diabetics in their bed complement. Such a ward allows the development of good teaching material used by experienced nursing staff. It also provides a focus of contact between patients and advice which may be obtained either by visit or by telephone. Greater experience of diabetes amongst the staff of such wards allows greater confidence both in staff and in patients. Thus, the staff-nurse on a diabetic ward will not think twice about allowing a patient to leave the hospital for a walk or to do some shopping, whereas for the staff of a busy medical ward such behaviour is alien to them and the feeling that the patient should be under their eyes all the time tends to persist.

Stablisation at home

The only real alternative to hospital admission is to consider stabilisation and education at home. A large staff are needed if this is to be undertaken but the costs of such staff have to be weighed against the costs of in-patient care. This system has been pioneered in England by the people at Leicester. Here, the diabetologist with the back-up of a number of health visitors and a dietitian undertake the stabilisation and education of young newly diagnosed insulin-dependent diabetic patients in their own home. This means teaching of the whole range of insulin injections and diet in the family context. It is generally felt that such a system has undoubted advantages over hospital admission. Emotively, the idea that the child is not taken away from the family or the home and learns in familiar surroundings is appealing. It must be said, however, that there is little evidence that home education is preferable to hospital education or vice versa. In support of either side of this argument comments from patients are often quoted. For example, a well-informed father of a diabetic boy commented after hearing the arguments for and against hospital admission of diabetic children 'my wife and I appreciated the time we had to ourselves while our son was in hospital', then went on to say that they were able to discuss how diabetes would affect them as a family and involve the other children in the preparations. What is more, they were able to express their hopes and fears openly without distressing the person at the centre of this upheaval. He was speaking in favour of a separation but undoubtedly his view was influenced by the fact that this was the method which he had experienced. Advocates of home education and stabilisation could quote similar stories in favour of home treatment. In making such comments there is no doubt that patients or their relatives are influenced by the system they have experienced.

Too much of the argument revolves around the newly diagnosed patient. Throughout this book we would like to stress that education is a continual process. Within this continual process are certain times when patients are perhaps more receptive. It is often advantageous to admit an adolescent or young adult who has passed from the care of a paediatrician to a physician. This allows assessment of the patient's knowledge of diabetes, a filling-in of any gaps that may exist, and hopefully good rapport between the patient and his new doctor.

What of the later years of life when patients may be changed from tablets to insulin? Here again, patients may be taught in their home about how to give their insulin injections. This is usually done by the district nurse and if this method is to be employed the supervising diabetic clinic really ought to ensure some degree of uniformity amongst their district nurses. Alternatively the patient may be brought up each day for a few days to learn the techniques involved. This is a useful method of teaching but does demand that staff are specifically allocated at certain times of the day to teach out-patients. Finally, we could admit these patients if the facilities were available. A few studies have been carried out comparing in-patient with out-patient care and management. It would be our impression that it often takes a considerably longer time to get the insulin dose approximately right if the patient is being stabilised as an out-patient. A young psychologist from a local university studied some of our diabetic patients who were being changed from tablets to insulin. We are in the fortunate position of having a small diabetic ward as our alternative to out-patient management. The findings of this young lady were interesting. She found that patients who had been admitted to the small diabetic ward had a better understanding of their condition and greater self-esteem than those patients attending the same unit on an out-patient basis. Similar and larger studies are of major importance before resources are committed on emotive grounds to either in-patient or out-patient care. The ideal situation, if there is one, might be to carry out the teaching of practical skills such as injection technique, urine or blood glucose testing etc., in the patient's own home, then to bring the patient together with others for the more theoretical aspects of diabetes. In this way better use might be made of local resources and the patients derive some benefit by sharing their experiences with others. The latter approach lends itself well to the teaching of non-insulin dependent patients. Group sessions within the hospital using the expertise of the dietitian, a chiropodist, a nurse and a physician work well and offer some education for the often neglected area of the non-insulin-dependent diabetic patient.

Preparing to teach the
    diabetic patient
Insulin injections
Blood glucose
    monitoring
Educating the
    teachers

5

Education of the diabetic patient

In the previous chapter we discussed the organisation of care for the diabetic patient both as an out-patient and an in-patient. Some of these situations, such as diabetic patients undergoing peritoneal dialysis or having a myocardial infarction, will not be met by the majority of nurses unless working in a speciliazed unit or during their training. We can now turn to situations where many nurses may well be called upon to play a major role in educating the diabetic patient. The two major demands for education in practical aspects of diabetic patient management are the teaching of insulin injections and of home-blood glucose monitoring. Other, no less important, aspects of education such as urine testing or dietary advice are covered elsewhere in this volume but teaching injection technique and blood glucose measurement are of such importance that they merit separate and extensive sections. We would do well to remember that good injection technique from the outset is a good investment for the insulin-dependent diabetic patient faced with the prospect of a life-time's daily ritual which may result in over 10 000 injections. In addition, bad habits which are imbued from the outset, such as failure to rotate injection sites, become increasingly difficult to break.

We should also remember that home blood glucose monitoring is an excellent means not only of improving diabetic control but of continuing education of the patient and is a means to greater knowledge, and confidence and ability to deal with the many different situations occurring in the life of the diabetic patient.

Few nurses or doctors are well equipped by their respective trainings to pursue a career as a teacher. Much of their ability is gained by experience, but experience does not necessarily grant greater insight into ways of approaching learning by the diabetic patient. For that reason, before dealing with these two important practical techniques, we should consider our approach to learning by the patient both from a psychological and from a practical stand-point.

PREPARING TO TEACH THE DIABETIC PATIENT

Introduction

It cannot be denied that the diabetic patient as a receiver of care is in a unique position. In no other medical condition is so much expected of the patient and of the patient's family. Self-management is essential for survival. To quote Dr R.D. Lawrence 'The diabetic patient must be his own doctor, dietitian, and laboratory technician. Hence education is the single most important aspect of treatment'. For too long this concept has been paid lip service only, but in recent years there has been an explosion of interest in the field of educating the diabetic patient. Writing recently, the President of the International Diabetes Federation, when comparing the many areas of advance in the treatment of diabetes, detailed as 'the most interesting development—and the fastest—is to be found in the areas of health care and information dissemination!' Yet, how well do we educate our patients? Do we plan our education, set out our aims and objectives and evaluate the success or failure of our teaching methods? How effective are we in motivating our patients, and do we influence longterm compliance? These are the questions nurses involved in patient education should be asking themselves.

The nurse educator, usually ill-prepared to tackle the problem, has to face the whole gamut of learning difficulties within her clientele: lack of motivation and apathy, wide variation of intellectual ability, age, emotional barriers and physical handicaps. Superimposed upon these problems may be the practical difficulties of limited time, inadequate space, and lack of teaching materials and equipment. Faced with all these problems we are still led to the conclusion that well-planned and executed patient education is not a luxury but a necessity.

What is learning?

Learning begins in utero and continues so long as the mind is active. It is influenced by numerous factors, genetic as well as environmental. Children often learn while not intending to, whereas certain forms of learning require a special effort on the part of the learner. Into the latter category fall desires to pass examinations, or to drive a car, or to be able to recognise a specific set of signs and symptoms and so diagnose diabetes mellitus. What have all these diverse learning situations in common? Basically it is that they lead to a change in behaviour. This allows us a definition of learning as 'a more or less permanent change in behaviour which is the result of experi-ence'. We may say that learning has occurred if we observe a change in behaviour. Applying this concept to the patient with diabetes mellitus learning to monitor their own blood glucose, the immediate and apparent change in behaviour would be the acquisition of a practical skill. A less immediate change would be the interpretation of the blood glucose levels and the adjustment of the insulin dose as a consequence of the results obtained. A more longterm change in the patient might be more self-confidence, better health care, and an increased sense of well-being.

Much of the research into the why and how of learning has been based largely on animal experiments. Much of the basis of the psychology of learning and its fundamental laws has been derived from the work of Pavlov, Thorndyke, and Skinner. It is not our intention to discuss their work in detail but a brief resumé is provided below since it is of considerable interest.

The Russian physiologist Pavlov was interested in the diges-tive system of dogs. He was led to his investigations by appre-ciation of the significance of his observations. Pavlov noticed that behaviour of dogs while being fed began to occur in expectation of being fed. This led to a series of experiments where the salivary duct in a dog's mouth was tapped and feeding of the dog was preceeded by a bell sounding. Repeatedly the bell/food sequence was presented to the dog. Gradually the amount of saliva produced began to increase as soon as the bell was sounded. This whole process was termed conditioning.

Working in America, Thorndyke placed a hungry cat into a cage with food outside the cage but visible through the bars. The pulling of a loop of wire or the pressing of a lever opened the door of the cage and allowed the animal access to the food. Initially it was noted that the cats indulged in wild and aggressive behaviour to get at the food. In the course of this behaviour the door would be opened by accident allowing the cat access to the food. If this experiment was repeated often enough the animal's behaviour shifted towards the vicinity of the door-opening mechanism. In addition, the period between being placed in the cage and getting out got progressively shorter. Eventually the cat would arrive at a position where having been put in the cage the escape mechanism would be operated immediately and food obtained.

A similar experimental device is the 'Skinner box'. This allows a particular piece of behaviour, for example pressing a lever or pushing a door open or pecking at a key, to be followed by a consequence such as the delivery of food or access to water.

This 'trial and error learning' has as one of its key concepts the idea of reinforcement. Transposing the experiments to the human situation one could liken this to rewarding a child with a sweet if the child has behaved well, but unless the reinforcement is sustained the change of behaviour, which is the result of learning, will fall off.

We would not wish the reader to think these simple learning situations are totally without interpretative problems. For further discussion of these the reader is referred to the book list at the end of this volume. One major concern must be whether these animal studies are really analogous to the human situation. Man has the advantage of language and complex ideas can be communicated through the spoken or written word. Reinforcement may be achieved by a job well done and indeed the knowledge that one has achieved a goal can be a potent reinforcer. It is essential that the learner has some feedback on his progress in order to sustain motivation. How does this apply to the diabetic patient? It does so by indicating the necessity for immediately reinforcing a correct response. A well-executed task such as drawing up of insulin correctly, or interpreting urine tests should be greeted by praise. The teaching session for the diabetic patient must be planned in such a way that the patient achieves the goal set out for him and this can only be done if a careful assessment is made of the patient's practical and cognitive skills at the beginning before any actual teaching is embarked upon. We should say that there is one exception to this rule and that is the first insulin injection. The patient is usually tense and afraid and it would be heartless to attempt any assessment before this first hurdle is overcome.

Educational aims and objectives

It is essential before embarking on any educational assessment to have one's aims and objectives firmly in mind. Many centres use a check list which can be ticked off, initialled and commented upon. We must not let this obscure the fact that each patient is different, their educational needs are different and will depend on age at diagnosis, level of intelligence, and motivation. In addition, the presence of physical or mental handicap and ability with language must be taken into account. As with the medical record, some form of documentation is absolutely necessary for accurate records and to chart progress. An example of such documentation is illustrated in Table 5.1a–c. This allows a guide to assessment, planning and evaluation of care and education.

Let us consider, firstly, the content of an educational programme. We may divide the content into three sets of information. There is a basic core of knowledge essential for survival, there is knowledge that the patient should know, and finally there is knowledge that the patient could know. How much is delivered to the patient for acceptance at any one time will be determined to a large extent by the experience of the nurse and a comprehensive assessment.

The diabetic patient needs to acquire certain practical and

Table 5.1a Assessment of the diabetic patient

Patient's understanding of his/her condition
Relatives' understanding of patient's condition
Patient/family reactions
Home conditions
Diet/nutrition
Recreation
Existing support services

Table 5.1b Physical assessment of the diabetic patient

Eyes and vision (visual acuity)
Skin
Mouth and dentition
Feet and circulation
Insulin injection sites

Table 5.1c Assessment and teaching of the diabetic patient

Psychomotor skills
Cognitive skills
Problems
Objectives
Evaluation

cognitive skills in order to survive. A 'survival package' is all that is required in the early days following diagnosis. Far too often the plethora of information is rained down upon the heads of the newly diagnosed patient and his family. This is not only futile and a waste of time but positively cruel, for how can a person who is stunned and distressed absorb, digest, and retain totally new concepts? Initial teaching must be simple and concise and broken down into small units which the patient can master and comprehend.

Acquiring a practical skill

Practical procedures such as the drawing up of insulin and the giving of the injection must be broken into a series of short steps. Each step should be talked through as well as demonstrated. Allow the patient to tell you in his own words, how he is going to perform this procedure as this is an excellent aid to memory. By using slides or a video it is possible to discuss

with the patient each step and the reasons why certain manoeuvres are carried out in a particular sequence. Elderly people, in particular, experience difficulty in acquiring a new skill
but with time, patience and appropriate teaching aids it is
possible to achieve success and to give this group of patients
a few years of independence. Elderly people serve as a good
example of why our educational aims must be clearly deline-
ated before commencing the educational programme. It must
be stressed that they do not cope very well when it comes to
drawing up two insulins in one syringe. For this reason pre-
mixed insulins such as Mixtard or Initard or a medium acting
insulin such as Monotard are preferable for this group of
patients.

When teaching patients practical skills remember to reinforce the desired behaviour of the time by 'well done, good,
that's right, etc.' and back-up your teaching by giving the
patient and their relatives educational literature which they can
read at their leisure.

In addition to insulin injection technique, a number of other
practical procedures form part of the survival package. These
include care of the equipment to be used and the procedure
for testing blood glucose or urine glucose.

Simultaneously with the teaching of these practical skills it
is necessary to cover some theoretical concepts. These are best
dealt with on a person to person basis using visual aids as well
as the spoken word, and the teaching augmented with
book/tape or slide/tape programmes or video cassettes.
Subjects which must be covered in these early days include
the avoidance or treatment of hypoglycaemia and hyperglycaemia, care during intercurrent illness, and the early introduction of ideas on diet.

Planning a teaching session

Define your objective which might be that the patient should
appreciate the effect of intercurrent illness on diabetic control
and be able to manage their diabetes during times of illness.

Try to relate to something the patient already knows.

Structure the material and deliver the most important information within the first ten to twenty minutes. Make sure that
the patient is following your train of thought by asking simple

questions and encouraging him to interrupt you if he does not understand.

Try to adhere to your brief and not be side-tracked unless it is relevant to the subject.

Finally, recapitulate emphasising all the salient points.

The advice given to new teachers is not out of place here, 'first of all you tell them what you are going to tell them, then you tell them, then you tell them what you have told them'. In order to reinforce the teaching and to assist the patient with consolidating information it is useful to refer them to relevant pages in patient education literature, or to a cassette so that the patient and his family can absorb the data in their own time and at their own pace. At the next teaching session it is advisable to ask straightforward questions relating to the previous session. In this way you are able to find out how much information has been imparted to the patient and his family and what is more important, how you have increased their overall understanding of diabetes. Remember the definition of learning—'a more or less permanent change in behaviour which is a result of experience'; also, there is a major difference between compliance and knowledge. A 98 per cent pass on a specially devised multiple choice question paper may tell you many things regarding the patient's knowledge and how effective you have been in communicating that knowledge to him. It does not, of course, indicate whether a change in behaviour will result from that knowledge—in other words, whether the patient is willing to comply with the information presented.

Practical points

Although we have discussed some aspects of patient education we have not considered where this should be done. Teaching in a hospital environment can have certain advantages over and against teaching within the home. A patient who is away from the pressures of the home must surely be in a more receptive state of mind. It is important to make the distinction between a quiet room set aside for teaching and the hurly-burly of a hospital ward. We have witnessed a patient being taught in a very small examination room, boasting one examination couch and one chair with no window and minimal ventilation. The patient had just been told by the physician that he had diabetes! The patient was seated on the one chair and the nurse was perched, somewhat inelegantly, on the examination couch. If the door was closed there was no air and if the door was left open the nurse had to compete with the noise from a busy diabetic clinic. There are one or two serious faults in this appalling situation—first of all, the cramped and claustrophobic environment; secondly, the position of the nurse seated inappropriately on the couch at a higher level than the patient looking down on him; and finally, the noise and distraction. We must consider the patient's reaction to this situation. Would this encourage him to think that he mattered as an individual? Does it appear that any trouble had been taken to provide a pleasant setting for this important encounter? it is a distressing reflection on the importance, or rather the lack of importance, we give the whole question of patient education. We doubt that this incident is uncommon but hopefully, with the increasing importance placed upon education of the patient, it will become a thing of the past.

A diabetic clinic is not an ideal learning place for the newly diagnosed patient and ideally all specific teaching should be carried out in a place set apart, be it in the patient's own home, in hospital, or in a health centre. As regards teaching in hospital, the nurse responsible for patient education must have a room in which to teach—this is not a luxury but a necessity.

Teaching material and equipment

We would do well as patient educators to ponder on the Chinese proverb 'I hear and I forget, I see and I remember, I do and I understand'. The first of these three statements implies that most people forget much of what they hear. It is certainly true that numberous studies have shown that the newly diagnosed patient will forget most of what is said to him by the nursing and medical staff. The patient selects what he wants to remember and the emotional shock which he is experiencing precludes any ability to absorb information other than that he has diabetes and that he needs to talk about it to his family and close friends. We must conclude from this that the spoken word alone has its limitations in patient education.

I see and I remember

So much of patient education can be enhanced by visual representation—urine testing, injection technique, foot care, blood glucose monitoring—the list is endless. Slides can be made by the good amateur photographer or ideally by the staff of the Clinical Illustration Department which should be available in most District Hospitals. Professionally produced synchronised tape/slide programmes are available for a modest sum from the British Diabetic Association and some similar educational material is available through the pharmaceutical industry. There are advantages in using home-produced slides as they represent exactly the technique taught in a particular unit. It is frustrating for the teacher and distracting for the patient to be told to ignore a particular section of a tape/slide programme simply because it does not reflect the current teaching in that particular centre. This drawback could be remedied at source by a greater degree of standardization in the teaching of practical procedures, particularly the insulin injection technique, throughout the country.

Films have a limited place in patient education. The equipment is heavy, costly and requires careful maintenance while the actual films are comparatively delicate.

Video-cassettes. Films have, to a large extent, been superceded by video-cassettes. There are many advantages with this versatile medium. A particular section of the video can be selected for discussion. The frame may be 'frozen' for a few minutes so that a relevant point can be emphasised. Most people are used to looking at a television screen and feel at ease with this medium. The cost is probably the greatest disadvantage and together with the need for a secure room in which to house the equipment. Unfortunately, there is no standardization of video-cassettes and it is important to ensure that one has the correct type for the receiver/players, or that facilities are available for the tape to be transfered from one system to another. In order to avoid violating copyright it is advisable to seek the permission of the maker. It is illegal to record television programmes which can infringe third party copyright but most television companies to date have ignored this if the material being recorded is for home use only.

Further legislation is being sought to stop the pirating of professionally produced material. We must remember that our patients are used to a high degree of professionalism in the commercially produced television programmes they see nightly on their sets. They will be irritated and distracted by amateurish productions however relevant they may appear to be to the teacher.

I do and I understand

The father of a diabetic made this comment 'We (the family) were told all about hypos, what we had to look out for, what we had to do, but it was only when we had to deal with it ourselves for the first time that we really understood what it was all about'. It is only through experience, and in this case the experience of living with diabetes, that the individual with diabetes or the parents of a diabetic child can come to any real understanding of the situation and make sense of the teaching they have received. This is exactly the same as learning a purely practical skill where the doing is the understanding.

Again, we return to the difference between knowledge and compliance, between learning what to do and actually doing it. Nurses are often irritated when the patient fails to make the correct response in a given situation. For example, a patient admitted with diabetic ketoacidosis may readily admit that diabetic control had been poor for four to five days prior to admission and yet had failed to take the appropriate action. Looking back through the patient record we might find that this very patient scored high marks when questioned about the causes, signs and symptoms, and treatment of diabetic keto-acidosis in the initial education and assessment. The patient knew what to do but did not do it, our gloom and despond-ency is complete.

Of course, there may be a good reason why this patient did not take steps to avoid the development of diabetic ketoaci-dosis. The commonest reason may be that patients were taught about diabetic ketoacidosis at the time of diagnosis but did not have to apply the knowledge that they gained until five or six years later. This brings us very clearly to the need for some form of continuing education.

Continuing education

It is primarily the newly diagnosed insulin-dependent diabetic patient who requires a survival package. Once this information that the patient needs to know has been communicated, a more leisurely approach to communicating what the patient should know and what the patient could know may be adopted.

With the non-insulin-dependent diabetic patient their survival package may simply be some simple modification of diet with or without an oral hypoglycaemic agent. That is not to imply that this much neglected group needs anything less in the way of education than the insulin-dependent diabetic patient. In similar manner, the two groups may be provided with information on a should and could know basis.

Continual educational courses and planned refresher courses would appear to be the acme of health education. Some centres in the United Kingdom are setting up refresher courses and the British Diabetic Association have established very successful educational weekends for the parents of diabetic children. Many centres in the United States of America, Australia, Canada and Switzerland have diabetic teaching centres to which patients, and in some cases their relatives, may go for a one or two weeks' refresher course. Patients may also be referred by other hospitals or by their family doctor. One such centre in Australia has a staff of seven, two nurses, two dietitians, two doctors and one social worker. The centre functions from 07.00 h to 17.00 h Monday to Friday and is open to patients and their relatives. The days are divided into a series of lectures, demonstrations, and discussion groups. Other centres have the added assistance of a psychologist who can help to identify those patients who may have more difficulty than most in accepting their disease and complying with the discipline diabetes imposes upon them. The presence of a psychologist in a discussion group where patients are encouraged to give verbal expression of their feelings helps to contain the discussion and give it a positive outcome. This type of educational centre can achieve an enormous amount of information dissemination. The diabetes education centre in Minneapolis has had more than four thousand patients through their educational programmes. In addition to the patients, over three thousand allied health professionals have attended for training and many have gone from there to begin their own training programmes in smaller hospitals and in the community.

In the United Kingdom resources are limited but there is little to prevent the sensible compromise of setting up regular single day refreshers for specific groups of patients. If classroom space within a hospital is limited a day of the weekend might be preferable and an enlightened catering officer may be persuaded to allow patients to take their midday meal in the staff canteen. Health visitors and community diabetic liaison nurses might have access to health centres with enough space for ten to twelve patients. While we cannot deal with the same numbers as our colleagues around the world and the facilities that we may be provided with do not bear comparison with theirs, the opportunities for patient education in the U.K. are there if the nursing, dietetic, chiropody and medical staff are sufficiently motivated and enthusiastic.

Group discussions or group therapy

One to one education is of course ideal but we must remember that if all our time is spent with individual patients we neglect the majority. Group discussions can circumvent this problem. Diabetic patients are rarely given an opportunity to discuss their feelings about being diabetic. The average exchange between patient and doctor in a diabetic clinic is purposely kept at a neutral level, partly because of time and partly because there is often no specific and tidy answer to many of the fears the patient might express. Group discussions might be the answer and help meet this need and could form an important part of the teaching programme. The diabetic team in Nottingham set up a discussion group which met weekly for a period of twelve weeks. The meeting was held in the evening and the group had their meal in the hospital canteen. The initial aims of the group are listed in Table 5.2. The organisers are to be applauded for attempting this venture. Inevitably mistakes were made and, importantly, have been learnt from. In retrospect, group organisers realised that the aims of the group should have been spelt out at the begin-

Table 5.2 Aims of discussion group

1. To give the participants an opportunity of getting to know other diabetics as people and thereby to reduce their existential loneliness.

2. Having an opportunity to express one's problems and frustrations in a supportive and non-judgemental atmosphere.

3. To get to know oneself as mirrored in other people's opinions.

4. To increase personal awareness.

5. To recognise that the ultimate responsibility rests with the individual no matter how much support and guidance is available from others.

ning as to what it could do and what it could not do. Specific rules were needed it was felt, with regard to the numbers attending, the length of sessions, and the number of meetings to be held. It must be emphasised that the group discussion is not an extension of the clinic and specific medical questions must not be raised. All the members must try to attend regularly and the proceedings must be confidential and should not be discussed outside the group. Splinter groups or mini-groups of two to three people discussing group business should be positively discouraged. Suggestions for the future include a series of short education sessions followed by discussion. While discussion in itself does not solve the problems it does help those taking part to approach their diabetes in a more positive way and with greater perspective.

INSULIN INJECTIONS

Insulin administration

With the discovery of insulin in 1921, it was possible for patients with insulin-dependent diabetes to live and pursue relatively normal lives. Few changes occurred in the mode of administration of insulin for over fifty years. Globin, zinc and protamine were added to regular insulin prolonging the duration of its action and porcine highly purified insulins, and then human insulin, were produced to reduce antibody formation. The actual injection of insulin by the subcutaneous route however, has remained unchallenged for decades.

Home blood glucose monitoring by patients and measurement of glycosylated haemoglobin has revealed the relatively poor control of many insulin-dependent diabetic patients. The importance of good control and attempts to obtain this has made physicians more aware of the way in which insulin is administered and when it is administered.

Subcutaneous injections

Syringes (Fig. 5.1)

The glass and metal syringes, 1 ml or 2 ml British Standard 1619, were introduced in 1954 and, to date, with the U100 glass and metal syringe, are the only syringes available on prescription in the United Kingdom. The syringe, together with a metal needle, 26 gauge, half inch, is stored in methylated spirit in a special carrying case. It must be emphasised that surgical spirit which contains castor oil and salicylic acid should not be used as the oil adheres to the syringe. Patients are advised to dismantle the syringe and carrying case and wash them in warm soapy water once a week. Careful rinsing and drying is

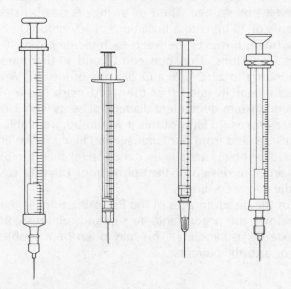

Figure 5.1 Syringes for insulin injection from left to right are:
2 ml British Standard 1619 U20 glass and metal needle
1 ml plastic syringe U20 with a fused needle
1 ml plastic syringe U20 with detachable needle
1ml British Standard 1619/2 U100 glass and metal needle.

important as rusting of the piston can occur. There is no need to boil the syringe to achieve sterility. There is even less need to boil the syringe, spirit and case as the father of one of our adolescent patients did recently.

U100 syringes

U100 insulin was introduced in the United Kingdom in 1983. The introduction of this strength of insulin had been planned for a number of years. Despite this planning, changing patients from U40 or U80 insulin to U100 insulin had to be spread over a period of two years. In part this was due to the inability of the manufacturers of glass and metal syringes to produce sufficient syringes. Two sizes of glass and metal syringes are available—1 ml and 0.5 ml (BS 1619/2) The 0.5 ml syringe has 50 divisions with one unit of insulin equivalent to one division on the syringe. Number of divisions and hence units of insulin are clearly marked in increments of 10 to a maximum of 50. Patients who require more than 50 units of insulin at one injection need a 1 ml syringe. The 1 ml syringe is clearly marked in increments of 10 units to a maximum of 100 units. Unlike the 0.5 ml syringe, however, between each increment of 10 there are only 5 divisions. Thus between 20 and 30 there are lines corresponding to 22, 24, 26 and 28 units of insulin. We must continually bear in mind that the word mark has a distinct meaning to insulin-dependent diabetic patients who used U40 and U80 syringes. In view of this it would be preferable if the word was deleted from our language in talking to patients.

The U100 syringes are slimmer and longer than the BS 1619 syringe and the design of the spirit proof carrying case has been adjusted accordingly.

One of the disadvantages of the BS 1619 syringe is that with continual use the piston tends to slip and requires considerable dexterity in handling. This may often be a problem for elderly or arthritic patients.

Plastic disposable syringes (Fig. 5.1)

Plastic syringes with a detachable or a fused needle have many advantages over the glass and metal syringes but regrettably are not available on prescription. The plastic syringe is light and easy to handle which is a major consideration for use with younger children and elderly patients. The piston is dependent and therefore less likely to slip when insulin is drawn up.

Considerable debate surrounds the word 'disposable'. The manufacturers of disposable syringes stress that the syringe be used once only. In practice many insulin-dependent diabetic patients use them for as long as the needle is good or if using a syringe with a detachable needle, for as long as the markings on the syringe are clearly visible. The syringes should be stored in a cool, clean place between injections. The occurrence of infection with repeated use of plastic disposable syringes appears to be minimal if it exists at all. Disposable equipment may be prescribed by physicians or paediatricians to certain patients and dispensed by the hospital pharmacy or clinic.

We should add that not all patients prefer plastic syringes and some indicate a clear preference for the glass and metal syringe. A number of patients opt to purchase disposable needles which can be used with the glass and metal syringe and stored in the carrying case.

Skin preparation

Clean, dry skin is all that is needed for a subcutaneous injection. A rub with an alcohol-impregnated swab achieves nothing and it is a waste of time and money. A certain mystique has grown up around the giving of an injection involving many unnecessary manoeuvres and a long list of basic requirements. Whether a patient is administering his own insulin or whether it is being administered by a nurse in the patient's home, a minimum amount of equipment is required.

    1 carrying case if using a metal or glass syringe
    1 syringe and needle
    1 or 2 bottles of insulin
    1 dry cotton wool swab (if absolutely necessary after slight blood loss)

Drawing up of insulin

It is important that patients are taught to inject air into the insulin bottle before drawing up the insulin, this prevents a vacuum forming and the slight increase of air pressure in the bottle assists the drawing up. Most patients experience some difficulty at first with holding the bottle and the syringe with one hand whilst manipulating the piston with the other. The 25 gauge, 5/8 inch and the 26 gauge, half-inch needles will support the weight of the insulin bottle so long as the syringe is held in the vertical position, leaving both hands free, one to hold the barrel of the syringe and the other to control the piston.

Drawing up a mixture of insulin

Many patients require a mixture of a short-acting insulin with a medium or long-acting insulin in a ratio which will vary according to their insulin requirements. Insulins are available with a fixed ratio of long to short-acting insulin which may be suitable for older patients or those controlled on a very small amount of insulin. But for the younger, more active patients, drawing up insulin from two separate bottles is the rule. Can all insulins be mixed? The answer is no. Species, purification, pH and manufacturer are relevant when mixing insulins. For example, Soluble Insulin B.P. is an older type of bovine insulin with a pH of 3.2, whereas Actrapid is a highly purified, porcine insulin, with a pH of 7. Both insulins are short acting but the acidity of the soluble insulin delays its absorption in comparison with the absorption and speed of action of the neutral actrapid. Examples of insulins which can be mixed include Neusulin and Neulente, Hypurin Neutral with Hypurin Isophane, Actrapid with Monotard, and Velosulin with Insulatard.

Mixing two insulins in one syringe

Procedure

1. Check insulins, e.g. expiry date, type and strength.
2. Gently rotate or invert the insulin bottles several times.
3. Inject air into the cloudy insulin bottle equivalent to the amount to be drawn up. Hold the bottle in the upright position so as to prevent the needle coming into contact with the insulin. Withdraw the needle.
4. Inject air into the clear insulin bottle and draw up the insulin

in the conventional way, ensuring that there are no air bubbles in the syringe.

5. Remove the bottle of clear insulin and replace with cloudy insulin and slowly draw down to the prescribed amount. If air bubbles are present at this stage, or too much insulin is inadvertently drawn up, then the insulin must be discarded and the whole procedure repeated.

It is important to draw up the 'clear' insulin first to avoid contamination with the 'cloudy' insulin. Contamination of short-acting insulin by longer-acting insulin will eventually alter its short acting properties.

Subcutaneous insulin injection technique (Fig. 5.2)

The angle at which an insulin injection is given is debatable. For many years the 45° angle has been favoured in the United Kingdom, but in the authors' opinion, the 90° angle is preferable for the majority of patients. After all, they are the consumers and their wishes should not be ignored. The 90° angle of insertion avoids the possibility of eventual intradermal injection and lessens the likelihood of palpable swellings occurring at the site of injection. When inserting a needle at 45° angle it is often necessary for the actual hold of the syringe to change to suit the site of the injection, whereas with the 90°

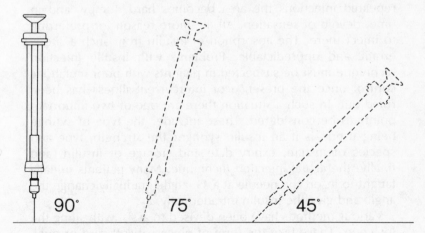

Figure 5.2 The angles of subcutaneous injections.

angle the 'hold' is the same and the insertion can be made rapidly, thus minimising the initial pain caused by puncturing the skin. Whether the skin is stretched or pinched up will depend on the fatness or thinness of the individual. Once the needle has been inserted it is unnecessary to withdraw the piston to see if the needle is in a blood vessel; if it is, there is no danger to the patient. The insulin should not be injected too rapidly as loss of insulin may occur if the needle is not firmly attached to the syringe, or if there is some blockage in the needle, the insulin therefore taking the line of least resistance. The patient is advised to wait a few seconds after injecting the insulin and withdrawing the needle as this appears to lessen the possibility of leaking from the puncture site. Occasionally there is blood loss from the site—firm pressure with a dry swab is all that is necessary. In some cases bruising will result, but patients should be assured all is well, unless, in rare circumstances, it occurs again and again.

Sites for insulin injection (Fig. 5.3)

Insulin given by a bolus subcutaneous injection can be injected in the following sites—upper arms, abdomen, the upper two-thirds of the thighs, buttocks, and some people even inject in the calves. Rotation of injection sites is important. Many children favour one particular site and with repeated injections the area becomes hard, lumpy, and in time, devoid of sensation. All the more reason for preferring to inject there. The absorption of insulin from such a site is erratic and unpredictable. Problems with insulin injection technique must be suspected in patients with poor metabolic control once the presence of intercurrent illness has been ruled out. In such a situation there are one or two important points to be considered. These include: the type of syringe being used—is it an insulin syringe? the strength, type and species of insulin, expiry date and storage of insulin, and finally, the actual injection technique. Many patients initially taught to insert the needle at a 45° angle gradually change the angle and give the insulin intradermally.

Various methods have been devised to assist with siting the injection. These take the form of pieces of soft card or polythene into which holes have been made at specified intervals. The card or polythene is placed over the site and the needle

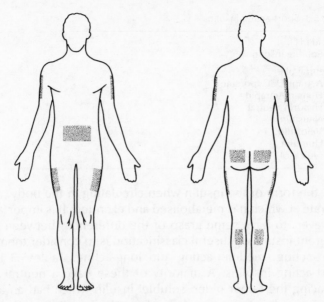

Figure 5.3 Sites for insulin injections.

inserted through the appropriate hole. In this way the whole area is used and one specific spot may not be injected for several weeks.

The absorption rate of insulin varies with type and site. Insulin is absorbed more rapidly from the abdomen compared with the thigh, and so it would appear to make sense to use this site in the morning, the aim being to try to lessen the rise of blood glucose after breakfast as this is usually the highest post-prandial peak of the day. In addition, absorption is more rapid from a shallow subcutaneous injection than a deep subcutaneous site.

Strenuous physical activity can effect insulin absorption, for example, riding a bicycle shortly after insulin has been injected into the leg, a phenomenon recognised by Dr Lawrence, himself an insulin-dependent diabetic. Hot baths after an injection can exert a similar effect.

Insulins

Although the insulin manufacturers specify times and duration of insulin action, this does, to some extent, vary with an individual depending upon rate of absorption from the injection

Table 5.3 Short-acting insulins

1. Acid pH
   Soluble insulin

2. Neutral pH
   Actrapid MC (porcine)
   Human Actrapid
   Hypurin neutral
   Neusulin
   Velosulin
   Humulin S
   Quicksol (100 u)

site, the form of the insulin when circulating in the body, and the rate at which it is metabolised and excreted. It is important, however, to have some grasp of the differences between the different insulins. A useful classification is to consider them as short-acting, medium-acting and long-acting. Table 5.3 lists short-acting insulins. A majority of these have a neutral pH replacing the rather older 'soluble' insulin which had an acid pH. Two advantages are claimed for the neutral solution in reducing the incidence of discomfort at injection sites and allowing more rapid absorption.

Medium-acting insulins or intermediate-acting insulin preparations are listed in Table 5.4. There are three major categories of intermediate-acting insulin preparations. Biphasic insulin injections are a mixture of beef insulin crystals in a

Table 5.4 Intermediate-acting insulin preparations

1. Biphasic
   Rapitard MC

2. Isophane insulins
   Isophane (NPH)
   Hypurin isophane
   Insulatard
   Neuphane
   Humulin I
   Monophane (100 u)

3. Zinc insulins
   Globin
   Semilente
   Semitard MC
   Monotard MC (porcine)
   Human Monotard
   Tempulin (100 u)

Table 5.5 Long-acting insulin preparations

Lente
Hypurin Lente
Lentard MC
Neulente
Ultralente
Ultratard MC
Protamine zinc insulin
Hypurin protamine zinc

solution of pork insulin. The two commonest ways of prolonging action of insulin, however, is to add protamine or zinc to an insulin preparation.

The intermediate-acting insulins are particularly appropriate for giving twice daily, mixed if necessary with short-acting insulins.

Long-acting insulin preparations are listed in Table 5.5. The majority of these are insulin zinc suspensions.

Strictly speaking, the lente family of insulins are mixtures having been derived originally from three parts of the amorphous form of insulin zinc suspension (semilente) and seven parts of the crystaloid suspension (ultralente). Much of the debate about whether insulins can be mixed derives from protamine zinc insulin which contains an excess of protamine unlike isophane insulin. A mixture of protamine zinc, with its excess of protamine, and soluble insulin results in conversion of the soluble insulin to more protamine zinc insulin in the syringe or in the subcutaneous injection site.

Not all of our patients can cope with drawing up a mixture of insulins. In these circumstances use of an insulin premixed by the manufacturer may be of value. Strictly speaking the lente family of insulins might be considered as 30/70 mixtures. In addition Mixtard insulin is a 30/70 mixture, neutral/isophane and Initard is a 50/50 mixture of neutral/isophane insulins.

Injection aids

The vast majority of insulin-dependent diabetic patients administer their own injections, and a person who has had diabetes 20 years may have given himself 15 000 injections. Most patients overcome the initial fear and abhorrence of injecting themselves, but a small minority cannot make that initial move to puncture the skin. Such patients could benefit by using an injection aid. There are two injection aids on the market:

a. The Palmer injector gun. This is a device which resembles a gun. The loaded syringe is slotted in position, the trigger is pulled and the needle is fired through the skin. The piston of the syringe is then depressed in the usual way.

b. Hypoguard automatic injector. This consists of two parts, a needle holder which fits on the BS1619 syringe, and a needle guard which is a small metal cylinder. It is important to note that the insulin must be drawn up through the needle holder to which a conventional needle is attached. Failure to do this will result in less insulin being given. The needle guard is placed over the needle and upper part of the needle holder. Pressure on the syringe springs the needle through the skin and the piston is depressed in the usual way.

There are advantages and disadvantages in both systems, but with the latter, the needle is obscured and the increased skin tension caused by the pressure of the needle guard further reduces the initial discomfort.

Injection aids for the visually handicapped

There are two insulin syringes designed specifically for blind or partially-sighted patients: a pre-set syringe and the click-count syringe. The pre-set syringe has a specially adapted piston which incorporates two screws. The larger screw adjusts the position of the piston and the smaller screw locks this in position. In practice this is not always the case and error in insulin dosage may occur. The disadvantage to the visually handicapped person is that the syringe must be set by a sighted person and checked regularly for accuracy.

The click-count syringe is designed in such a way that the two senses, hearing and touch, are utilised. An audible click and a notch in the piston are equivalent to one mark on the syringe. This allows much more independence and error is lessened. Nevertheless, it is strongly recommended that the patient be instructed and observed using the syringe by a member of the medical or nursing profession. With constant use and wear and tear the click may become less distinct and therefore the syringe will need replacing at regular intervals. Although the manufacturer suggests that two insulins may be drawn up with the click-count syringe, it is certainly not recommended for every patient. Independence must be weighed against safety and good metabolic control. The nurse or physician must decide, with the patient and, if possible, with the patient's family what each is trying to achieve. It may be that a degree of independence must be forfeited for the sake of an improvement in blood glucose levels.

Insulin-bottle location jig

The plastic location jig is useful for the visually handicapped and for those with a tremor who find it very difficult to locate the rubber cap of the insulin bottle. An ingenious device has recently been developed by a plastic syringe manufacturer, which incorporates a location jig and a magnifier, which magnifies the marks on the syringe $2\frac{1}{2}$ times (Fig. 5.4). Some of the aids listed above are not available on prescription but can be provided at the discretion of a hospital physician. Perhaps a word or two about the Drug Tariff would not be out of place here. Drugs, equipment and applicances which can be prescribed by general practitioners are listed in the Drug Tariff, published by The Department of Health and Social Security and amended at regular intervals. The initial cost of drugs and equipment etc. is met by the individual pharmacist who purchases his stock through a wholesale chemist. The dispensed prescriptions are then forwarded to a government agency for financial reimbursement. The pharmacist who inadvertently dispenses a drug or equipment which is not listed in the Drug Tariff must meet the entire cost himself. Hospital pharmacists vary enormously as to what they are prepared to provide, or able to provide. Within certain financial constraints, for example, it may be possible to provide all the initial therapy a newly diagnosed patient requires but to set some limitations on the dispensing of blood glucose strips for patient home blood glucose monitoring. Some might argue that it is preferable to prescribe the syringes and needles for dispensing via retail pharmacists, thus making more money

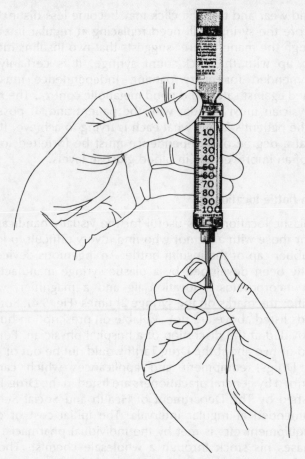

Figure 5.4 Insulin-bottle location jig and magnifier (Becton-Dickinson).

available in the hospital pharmacy for blood glucose strips. It can only be a matter of time before blood glucose strips are available on prescription, making such decisions unnecessary.

Complications of insulin injections

Local allergic reactions

Very occasionally local allergic reactions at injection sites can arise. The patient usually complains of burning and itching of the skin and redness following injection. In the majority of cases it is transitory and the patient should be reassured that it will pass. Calamine can be applied locally or an anti-histamine prescribed if necessary. It may be sensible to change the manufacturer or the species of insulin although this does not always result in loss of the allergic reaction.

Lipoatrophy

Lipoatrophy occurs mainly in women and is a wasting of subcutaneous fat at or near injection sites. It gives rise to unsightly pits and hollows and at its worst may preclude a young girl from wearing a bikini. The problem is considerably less with the highly purified insulins which most of our patients now use. Patients who remain on the old soluble and isophane insulins should be questioned specifically about hollows at injection sites and when these occur it is sensible to change the patient to a more recently introduced insulin.

The underlying reason for the atrophy is unclear but is probably a local immune response. It should go without saying that when lipoatrophy occurs the patient's injection technique should be checked.

Lipohypertrophy

As the name implies this condition is the exact opposite of lipoatrophy. With lipohypertrophy there is an increase in subcutaneous fat at or near the injection site. This may be severe with a large pad of fat seen in the upper thighs, particularly in women. Again, embarrassment may ensue if the patient wishes to wear shorts or a swimsuit.

The cause is unknown but it does not appear to be related to immune mechanisms since the incidence has not decreased with the introduction of highly purified insulins. Invariably it is associated with poor injection technique, particularly failure to rotate injection sites. With continual use of one site an insensitive area of skin comes to overlie an equally insensitive fat pad. Patients should be encouraged to alter their injection sites but disappearance of the fat pad is rarely quick.

Infection

Infection at injection sites is extremely rare and there is some anecdotal evidence of farmers injecting insulin through their trousers. While we would not necessarily condone this procedure it does illustrate the point made earlier that ordinary cleanliness is quite sufficient prior to injection and that a wipe with an alcohol swab is a waste of time and money.

Insulin antibodies

In 1956 insulin antibodies were identified in the serum of insulin-treated diabetic patients. The significance of insulin antibodies in the treatment of diabetes has never been completely clarified. At various times suggestions have been made that insulin antibodies are associated with the development of longterm diabetic complications or that transplacental transfer of antibodies might be harmful to the foetus of the diabetic mother. None of these claims have been substantiated. It must be remembered, however, that both beef and porcine insulin are foreign proteins to a human being. It is not surprising, therefore, that some degree of immune response is elicited over the course of the many thousands of injections a diabetic patient may receive. It is quite clear, following the introduction of highly purified insulins, that much of the antibody production which was provoked by older insulins was due to a lack of purity in the insulin. Antibody production in response to highly purified porcine insulin is minimal. Similarly, we might expect that antibody response to human insulin would be rare if it occurred at all. Low titres of antibodies do indeed occur to human insulin and highly purified porcine insulin although it remains unclear whether the antibodies are produced in response to the agent added to the insulin to prolong its action, rather than to the purified chemical insulin itself.

BLOOD GLUCOSE MONITORING

Blood glucose monitoring by the patient in the home was introduced as early as 1962 when Doctors Keen and Knight had certain patients taking capillary blood samples on to filter papers which were then passed to a hospital laboratory for analysis. This had the obvious disadvantage that the method did not give instant results but it did reveal the poor control of most of the patients who took part in the project.

In 1970 the Ames Company produced a single 'solid phase' system—glucose oxidase strips used with a reflectance meter. With the introduction of battery operated machines and, more recently, of semi-quantitative strips which can be used without a meter, patients can now carry out blood glucose estimations almost anywhere and at any time.

Technique

Capillary blood is easily obtained from the pulp of the fingers and thumbs. The skin should be clean and free from sweat. Most patients prefer to use Monolet lancets with or without a spring-loaded gadget (Fig. 5.5). With all of the sticks in current use it is important that a good size drop of capillary blood be applied to the test patch (Fig. 5.6). Obtaining and applying a drop of blood to the reagent stick is similar regardless of the

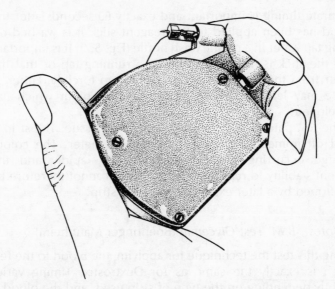

Figure 5.5 Obtaining capillary blood with an Autolet (Owen-Mumford).

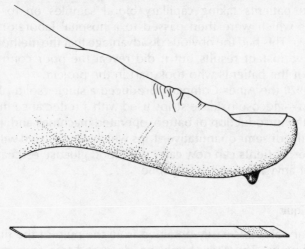

Figure 5.6 Applying the blood to a reagent stick.

type of strip. With different sticks, however, there are slight differences in the subsequent procedure.

Dextrostix (Ames)

Accurate timing is important and exactly 60 seconds after the blood has been applied to the reagent stick it is washed off using tap water in a plastic wash bottle (Fig. 5.7). It is important that the stick is not washed under a running tap or that the water from the wash bottle be applied too forcibly. Either of these may lead to a leaching out of the colour which has developed.

The test patch is then blotted with a soft tissue. The strip is read off immediately in the appropriate meter. The colour change occurring with Dextrostix fades rapidly and the patient's ability to report accurate results cannot therefore be confirmed by a later examination of the strip.

Reflotest, B.M. Test Glycemie (Boehringer Mannheim)

Using this test the technique for applying the blood to the test patch is exactly the same as for Dextrostix. Timing varies slightly depending on the type of strip used, and the blood is wiped off the test patch with a cotton wool swab (Fig. 5.8). The

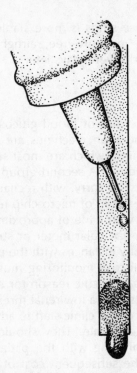

Figure 5.7 Washing surplus blood from a reagent stick (Dextrostix-Ames).

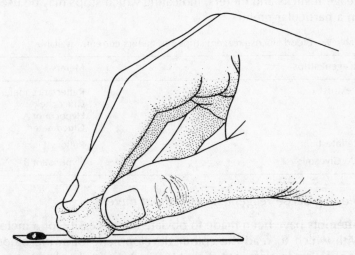

Figure 5.8 Wiping surplus blood from a reagent stick (BM Test glycemie-Boehringer Mannheim).

colour change on these strips is more stable and so long as they are stored in a moisture-free, airtight container, the results can be checked several days later.

Blood glucose meters

There are three main types of blood glucose meters on the market. The first generation machines are mains operated, somewhat bulky machines which are most suitable for use in hospitals or health centres. A second group of machines are more compact and easy to carry, with rechargeable batteries. The third group is the result of micro-chip technology; these meters have batteries with a life of approximately 1000 blood tests. The choice of a particular meter or strip may rest with the physician or in many instances with the patient. The costs of long-term blood glucose monitoring must be met by the patient unless there is a specific reason for blood testing, for example those patients with a low renal threshold to glucose. It is the responsibility of the clinic staff to advise on the types of meters and strips available. They should also be aware, when discussing monitoring with the patient, of the initial financial outlay and the subsequent cost of strips and maintenance of the machines. Table 5.6 lists the currently available reagent sticks and meters, indicating which strips may be used in a particular meter.

Table 5.6 Blood glucose reagent strips and meters currently available

Reagent strips	Meters
Dextrostix	Reflectance meter
	Glucochek
	Hypocount A
	Glucometer
Reflotest	Reflomat
BM Glycemie	Hypocount B

Blood glucose reagent sticks without meters

Attempts have been made to obviate the necessity for a meter with which to read the colour development following blood application to a reagent stick. Most experience has been accumulated using B.M. Glycemie 20–800, although a second, similar stick has been introduced recently. Both B.M. Glycemie 20–800 (Boehringer Mannheim) and Visidex (Ames) have two separate reagent pads which develop two different colours. One colour is more suitable for reading low blood glucose concentrations and the other more suitable for reading high blood glucose concentrations. Once developed, the colours are stable and may be read at a later date. This allows the nurse to check the accuracy of the patient's reading of the colour even when the test was done days previously in the home.

Why should patients do blood glucose monitoring?

It does not take an intelligent patient long to realise that there are discrepancies between how he feels and the results of urine tests. Urine tests do not necessarily reflect the prevailing blood glucose concentration. Studies with diabetic children at a summer camp demonstrated that a negative urine test could be associated with blood glucose estimations ranging from 2.2 to 10 mmol/1. The normal renal threshold for glucose is 10 mmol/1 but there are individual variations. This fact is often ignored. With the aid of blood glucose monitoring it is possible to assess the patient's renal threshold without hospital admission. A study in Nottingham of 47 insulin-dependent patients carrying out blood glucose and urine testing demonstrated that the renal threshold to glucose varied considerably in some instances by as much as 3 to 12 mmol/1. There is also a wide range of increments in blood glucose concentration which will change a urine test from negative to 2 per cent. In some patients this range is as small as 2 to 4 mmol/1 yet in others an increase of as much as 12 to 15 mmol/1 is needed to span the change in urine glucose.

A further problem which the patient encounters in interpreting urine tests is how negative is a negative test? If the renal threshold is 10 mmol/1 a negative urine test may indicate that the patient's blood glucose is within the normal range but it will not distinguish between a normal blood glucose and a blood glucose in the hypoglycaemic range. Small wonder that the patient derives little comfort from this. If our patient has an elevated renal threshold for glucose, however, a negative urine test may occur with the blood glucose in the normal range, hypoglycaemic, or hyperglycaemic.

While these criticisms of urine testing are well founded we are not attempting to make a case for the abolition of urine testing. The vast majority of diabetic patients do test their urine, and will continue to do so in the foreseeable future. We should also make the point that it is possible still to make adjustments of insulin doses on the basis of urine tests. In addition, for the non-insulin-dependent diabetic patient urine tests remain a reasonable guide to blood glucose control.

When to test and how often

One temptation for the diabetic patient who has recently learned how to measure his own blood glucose is for him to do the test at all hours of the day and night. This produces a large number of results but the interpretation of these results may be difficult in view of the random timings. It is better to advise patients to carry out four pre-prandial blood estimations on two consecutive days per week. We must recall that measurement of blood glucose concentration is not an end in itself but is a means to the end of adjusting insulin doses to improve diabetic control. Thus there is a clear responsibility when teaching patients how to measure their blood glucose in the home, also to give them clear instructions on how to interpret the results obtained and the action to take in the adjustment of their therapy. For the intelligent patient adjustment of insulin dosage based on blood glucose levels may well be easy. They may have a good grasp of the time course of action of the insulins which they give themselves. The majority of patients, however, will need some constant reminder of the steps they should take in response to a particular pattern of tests. Some patients prefer written guidelines while others are reassured by telephone contact with clinic or ward staff. It is important to stress that the nurse who advises the patient on changes of insulin dose should never simply listen to the patient's blood test results and then reel off a new insulin dose, but should always ask the patient what adjustment of insulin the patient feels should be done in response to a particular set of results. It is only in this way that the patient will gain confidence in their own ability to alter their insulin therapy without constant recourse to professional advice. In other words, even the telephone call by the patient is a means by which the nurse can offer further education on specific points. Once reasonable control of blood glucose has been achieved by this means the patient may then progress to measurement of post-prandial blood glucose and, if necessary, further insulin adjustments can be made on the basis of these results.

Blood glucose monitoring in special situations

There is no doubt amongst nurses and physicians that patient blood glucose monitoring is an excellent educational tool. Many patients speak with confidence about their pre and post-prandial blood glucose levels and are considerably more aware of the duration of insulin action, while having greater confidence in their ability to adjust insulin doses.

Pregnancy and blood glucose monitoring

In recent years there has been a great improvement in the outcome of pregnancy in diabetic women (Ch. 6). Previously, pregnancy in an insulin-dependent diabetic patient was associated with a high morbidity and mortality of the foetus. The ability of obstetricians to monitor the growth and development as well as the wellbeing of the foetus has contributed significantly to this improvement. It is also generally accepted that the attention of the physician to improving and maintaining good diabetic control has been of major importance. Such was the accent upon good diabetic control during the last trimester of pregnancy that it became standard practice to admit insulin-dependent diabetic women at this time. This meant that the pregnant diabetic patient might spend a considerable proportion of her pregnancy in hospital. While this may have been feasible for the women having her first baby, it created considerable difficulties for the mother with one or more children at home.

Blood glucose monitoring has made it possible for good diabetic control to be achieved at home. This means that excluding obstetric complications, patients may now be admitted later in their pregnancy and some centres would not advocate admission in an uncomplicated pregnancy until 38 weeks. The number and frequency of the blood tests is decided by the physician and the patient, but we should not make excessive demands upon our patients. The pregnant woman is usually highly motivated and has a definite goal. She will do many things to ensure a successful outcome to her pregnancy but it is all too easy to take advantage of her motivation and demand vast numbers of home blood glucose tests. A reasonable compromise reached in many centres is to require of the patient 7 to 10 tests a day for 2 days each week. This allows pre-prandial and post-prandial assessment of blood glucose concentration as well as the important test in the early hours of the morning when it is well recognised that hypoglycaemia may go unrecognised by the patient.

Diabetic control during conception. The marked reduction in recent years of perinatal deaths is not reflected in a similar reduction in the incidence of congenital malformations in young insulin-dependent diabetic women who are pregnant. Major malformations remains two to three times more common in the infants of women who have diabetes at the time of conception (Ch. 6). There is tentative evidence that malformations may be related to poor diabetic control at conception and in the early weeks of pregnancy when foetal organs develop. In view of this good metabolic control prior to, and at the time of conception is advocated. Pre-conception counselling should be available for all diabetic women of child-bearing age and form part of the diabetic education of adolescent girls. At this time it is wise to implant the idea that good diabetic control is important around the time of conception, into the woman's mind. We should not be prepared to do this however, unless at the same time we can give her a means of improving metabolic control. Home blood glucose monitoring is extremely useful in this context and should be introduced at this stage.

Nocturnal hypoglycaemia

It is perhaps true to say that urine testing for glucose is at its most valueless to the patient at bedtime. Obtaining a negative urine test at this time, as encouraged by the physician, may generate a real fear of hypoglycaemia while asleep. This fear is very real in children who readily confess that they are afraid of hypos while asleep and not waking up in the morning. The measurement of blood glucose concentration at this time may considerably allay these fears.

Certain patients are particularly susceptible to nocturnal hypoglycaemia. These include the pregnant diabetic patient and the brittle diabetic patient.

In 1953, Somogyi described rebound hyperglycaemia following a hypoglycaemic episode. Traditionally, this has been attributed to stimulation of release of counter-regulatory hormones by hypoglycaemia. The release of adrenalin, glucagon, and corticosteroids not only corrects the hypoglycaemia but may drive the blood glucose into the hyperglycaemic range. Thus when hypoglycaemia occurs during sleep and is counteracted by this surge of counter-regulatory hormones, the patient may awaken with heavy glycosuria. To an unsuspecting doctor this implies that the evening dose of long-acting insulin should be increased in order to prevent early morning hyperglycaemia. This, of course, is exactly the wrong treatment. The raised blood glucose in the morning has occurred because of a hypoglycaemic episode during the night and the correct treatment, therefore, would be to abolish the hypoglycaemic episode by a reduction in insulin dosage. That hypoglycaemia occurs during the night may be documented by the patient's home blood glucose monitoring. If very careful explanation of this suspicion is made to the patient many will be only too happy to set the alarm for 2.00 or 3.00 am and, on wakening, measure their blood glucose.

We should just add that the Somogyi phenomenon or rebound hyperglycaemia is a phenomenon whose existence is doubted by some. Nevertheless it is clear when home blood glucose monitoring is done in the early hours of the morning that a number of our patients do indeed have blood glucose levels in the hypoglycaemic range at this time. While any accompanying symptoms may be insufficient to wake the patient from sleep we cannot be absolutely sure that repeated nightly hypoglycaemia is not harmful to these patients.

Changes in insulin regimens

Changing from one injection of insulin a day to two injections can be managed as an out-patient. The procedure is considerably helped by home blood glucose monitoring by the patient. The patient should be advised to carry out four pre-prandial blood glucoses per day, and with adequate guidelines most patients can adjust their insulin therapy. Alternatively, telephone or direct contact with the community liaison nurse may prove most supportive at this time.

An educational tool

From the foregoing it is readily apparent that teaching patients the technique of home blood glucose monitoring, the interpretation of their results, and the action that should be taken in response to particular patterns make a significant contribution to the expansion of the patient's knowledge about their diabetes. In view of this, it is not surprising that the benefits of the technique of home blood glucose monitoring cannot be separated from the benefits of enhancing the patient's knowledge. In many studies of home blood glucose monitoring, insufficient attention has been paid to the educational aspect. In one of the best studies in Newcastle upon Tyne, 46 insulin-dependent patients on twice daily injections were studied during traditional urine tests, blood glucose measurements with strips and a meter, and blood glucose measurements using strips alone. Before the strips were introduced into the study there was an initial run-in period of 6 months during which the three groups based their control on urine testing. During this time the patient received intensive education, attending a special clinic every 2 weeks and seeing one of two doctors for 30 minutes per visit. In addition, there was direct access by telephone. After this initial educational period there were three month crossover periods. The results were most interesting, indicating a most significant improvement in control (assessed by glycosylated haemoglobin measurement) during the educational period which was not improved upon after blood glucose monitoring was introduced. In a more modest study comparing two groups of insulin-dependent diabetic patients, one group using urine testing and the other home blood glucose monitoring in an attempt to improve diabetic control, we found a modest improvement in diabetic control in both groups implying little benefit from home blood glucose monitoring alone. Despite these findings, when patients are considered for study purposes as groups, few people would deny that individual patients may have their lives revolutionised by home blood glucose monitoring.

The point we would wish to make is the difficulty in separating the technique and the education of the patient which is involved during the teaching of the technique. In other words the effect of education on diabetic control cannot be ignored or, more specifically, the interest and the time taken with the individual patients. In both the above studies a great deal of time was given to the patients and other aspects of their diabetes were undoubtedly influenced. For example, more attention was probably paid to diet and in some instances to overall health care. As the rapport between patient and nurse or patient and doctor improved, psycho-social problems were discussed and more and more time was given over to counselling and less to the actual monitoring. This is not to deny the advantages of blood glucose monitoring but to emphasise the need for regular follow-up of patients, with reinforcement and with continuing two-way discussion on diabetic control and factors which influence this, including adjustment of insulin dosage.

Other effects of home blood glucose monitoring

Only a few psychological studies of patients undertaking blood glucose monitoring have been carried out. One of these of interest is the report from the Department of Psychiatry at Cornell University when young adult, insulin-dependent patients were studied. Psychological assessment was made before and during an intensive programme of self-monitoring of blood glucose. It was found that initially the patients were bewildered and resisted passively to the demands of the programme. It was also found that at the outset all patients appeared depressed, as demonstrated by a high score on the Hamilton rating scale which is a psychological test for assessing the degree of depression. During the course of the programme the emotions of anger, resentment and fear gave way to better self-reliance, diminished anxiety and better acceptance of their illness. After 8 months there was an appreciable improvement in the Hamilton rating scale. All ten patients had improved diabetic control and were less depressed. This study would appear to suggest that blood glucose monitoring with better metabolic control leads in turn to an improvement in emotional wellbeing. As a rider to this, perhaps we should add that interest in individual patients was probably extremely important since, as we have hinted above, success in improving diabetic control may well be commensurate with the amount of time spent with the patient.

EDUCATING THE TEACHERS

It is appropriate at the end of this chapter that some thought is given to the training of the teachers. In this context the establishment of a grade of 'Clinical Nurse Specialist' within the nursing career structure is to be welcomed. The clinical nurse specialist in diabetes has, as a major part of her job, education of the patient. In addition it is likely that she will play a significant role both in pre-registration nursing education and in the training of more senior colleagues. This being so, we must consider whether holders of these positions should be given some specialist training in diabetes. The alternative would appear to be that further education in the subject should be entirely by chance or through extensive experience.

It remains to be seen how many of these posts will be established within the National Health Service. There are a number of specialties which quite clearly would benefit from such posts. This means that the establishment of a clinical nurse specialist in diabetes will have to compete for funding with these other specialties and it is thus unlikely that any centre in the U.K. will have a staff complement to match diabetes centres in the U.S.A. or Australia or the rest of Europe (p. 182). The task of both primary or continuing education of the patient as well as education of junior colleagues will continue, therefore, to fall on the holders of a multitude of nursing posts. These include the out-patient staff, ward staff, and community staff. Thus, the ward sister teaching a patient the technique of insulin injections and accompanied by a junior nurse should be aware that the teaching of the nurse and of the patient are proceding simultaneously. It is a source of gratification to all members of the health care-team caring for diabetic patients that there has been an explosion of interest within the nursing profession in diabetes. This is readily apparent from organised study days or from specialist courses specifically for nurses. Recently, acknowledgement of the demand for higher training in diabetes has come from the Joint Board of Clinical Nursing Studies with their recognition of a course in diabetes (Course No. 928). The aim of this course is to enable registered nurses and state certified midwives to study new developments and update their skills and knowledge of the care and management of diabetic patients, and importantly, including teaching and counselling. Our own course in Birmingham, which is approved by the Joint Board of Clinical Nursing Studies actually predates the formal establishment throughout the country of a diabetes course. The Birmingham course which was established in 1978 takes the form of a day-release course over twenty weeks. Teaching is given through formal lectures, discussions, ward rounds and some project work. Through links with other hospitals in the city the participants have been able to see at first hand the treatment of patients with diabetic retinopathy, the care of the pregnant diabetic woman, and the special problems posed by caring for children with diabetes. Clearly, since the course is a day-release course there are geographical constraints upon attendance. If, as is hoped, more centres accept the responsibility of establishing a Joint Board Course this limitation will disappear.

As an entirely separate venture we have held residential courses for trained nurses interested in diabetes. Participants have been drawn from nursing staff, not only from the UK and the Republic of Ireland but from other parts of Europe. A feature of each course has been a demand for places which far exceeded the number of participants which we felt was ideal. Importantly, participants have come from both the community and the hospital and have included among the latter, nurses from obstetric and paediatric wards. We have regularly resisted the temptation to accept predominantly teaching hospital nurses, feeling that the nurse working on her own in a district general hospital might receive most benefit from the course.

One of the major problems with the residential course, which it must be hoped will not influence the Joint Board of Clinical Nursing Studies course, has been the difficulty nurses have experienced in obtaining funding. Financial arrangements for post-registration nurse training differ greatly from region to region. It is a source of regret that a few intended participants have been refused any contribution to either their expenses or the course fees by their employing authority. Fortunately, the British Diabetic Association and the pharmaceutical industry have been considerably more receptive when such difficulties have arisen.

We feel that post-registration nursing training in diabetes is of immense importance. Centres with facilities for the establishment of a recognised course should be cajoled or badgered into setting this up. There can be little doubt that investing time in the education and training of nursing staff will reap rich rewards in the standard of care of diabetic patients.

6

Care of the diabetic patient in special situations

PREGNANCY AND CONTRACEPTION

Pregnancy worsens the metabolic control of established diabetes and any tendency to diabetes may be brought to light during pregnancy. Poor metabolic control is associated with a poor outcome and good metabolic control plays a vital part in ensuring a satisfactory outcome. The results of pregnancy complicated by maternal diabetes are directly proportional to the efforts made by the patient and the combined medical, obstetric and neonatal team. Unlike the long-term aspects of diabetes, the results of diabetic management in pregnancy can be measured easily for example in terms of perinatal mortality, congenital malformations, infant birth weight and hypoglycaemia. Many of the metabolic changes in pregnancy are important for diabetes. In the normal subject there is an increase in stimulated insulin secretion even in the early stages of pregnancy, and this may be one of the factors that helps to increase the maternal fat stores in early and mid gestation. In late pregnancy the ratio of serum insulin to blood glucose level almost doubles. Basal insulin concentrations are normal in the first and second trimester but are increased in the third trimester. The effectiveness of insulin to reduce blood glucose is impaired progressively as pregnancy proceeds. The precise cause of this relative insulin resistance is unknown though counter-regulatory hormones such as glucagon, sex steroids and cortisol are elevated and the placental lactogen hormone has similar diabetogenic effects to growth hormone. Measurements of insulin binding to cell receptors in human pregnancy have not shown any consistent abnormality, so it is likely that part of the insulin resistance is due to changes in the post-receptor response to insulin (Ch. 2).

Pregnancy in the normal subject results in a reduction in fasting blood glucose concentrations of up to 1 mmol/l in late gestation. The lower fasting blood glucose level may be due to the relatively high insulin to glucagon concentration reaching the liver which restrains glucose output by the liver, and at this stage the fetus is also using maternal glucose as an energy fuel. Oral and intravenous glucose tolerance tests, on the other hand, show a relative intolerance to glucose developing in the third trimester. There is an increase in the peak glucose concentration of approximately 1 mmol/l and a prolongation of hyperglycaemia after oral glucose. Studies of diurnal blood glucose profiles in normal pregnancy, however, have not shown any changes in mean blood glucose levels while eating normal meals, though the range of blood glucose tends to be greater as pregnancy progresses. Another important physiological change that occurs during pregnancy is a lowering of the renal threshold for glucose. This occurs fairly early in pregnancy and is probably due to an increase in the filtration rate through the kidney. Glycosuria poses two problems, the detection of diabetes is made more difficult when renal glycosuria is relatively common, and monitoring of established diabetes in pregnancy by urine testing may be misleading.

Pregnancy also has important effects on fat metabolism. When glucose is not available during starvation fat can be mobilised quickly and ketone body production accelerated (Ch. 1). After overnight starvation plasma non-esterified fatty acid and ketone body concentrations are normal but with more prolonged starvation or with poor carbohydrate intake levels rise. Whether hyperketonaemia is harmful to fetal growth and development is uncertain.

Problems in pregnancy complicated with maternal diabetes

Maternal fertility is normal and there are no particular maternal risks during pregnancy, providing suitable adjustments to therapy are made to ensure adequate metabolic control. Pregnancy has no permanent effect on diabetic control, the therapy needed after delivery is usually similar to that before conception. The chronic complications of diabetes are mostly unaffected by pregnancy. Occasionally established retinopathy may deteriorate in pregnancy and require laser or photocoagulation treatment. Whether such deterioration would have occurred anyway in that particular individual, or whether pregnancy had a specific effect cannot be proven. It is of course hoped that strict metabolic control achieved in pregnancy will go some way towards preventing the development of chronic complications.

1. First trimester

The excess of major congenital malformations that is found in the infants of insulin-dependent diabetic mothers has drawn attention to the importance of metabolic control in the first few weeks after conception. It is likely that some aspect of poor diabetic control is a factor in causing these malformations. Spontaneous abortion has not been shown to occur any more frequently in diabetic patients compared with the non-diabetic population, but poor diabetic control may contribute to abortions.

2. Second trimester

Less is known about the effects of maternal diabetes in this stage of pregnancy. Initially fetal growth as judged by ultrasound scanning tends to be a little delayed but is usually normal later.

3. Third trimester

One of the greatest fears in the management of pregnancy in a patient with diabetes is the problem of sudden stillbirth occurring in the 2–3 weeks before term. The cause of most of these stillbirths is unknown but is usually associated with poor or indifferent metabolic control. There is no doubt that an episode of severe ketoacidosis in the mother is associated with approximately 50 per cent fetal loss. On the other hand no firm evidence can be found that clinical hypoglycaemia in the mother has any deleterious effect on the fetus at any stage during pregnancy.

4. The neonate

The classic infant of the mother whose diabetes has been poorly controlled is obese, plethoric and sleepy. Such an infant feeds poorly and is subject to hypoglycaemia. The birth-weight is greater than the 90th centile corrected for gestational age due mainly to an increase in body fat. This increase in birth weight may result in difficulties in vaginal delivery with resulting birth trauma. During pregnancy glucose freely crosses the placenta to the fetus but maternal insulin does not. If, in a diabetic woman, blood glucose is raised then fetal glucose will stimulate insulin secretion by the fetus. At birth the withdrawal of maternal glucose supply will result in hypo-glycaemia because preceding high maternal and fetal blood glucose levels caused beta cell hypertrophy in the fetal pancreatic islets and excessive insulin secretion. The tendency to hypoglycaemia is also brought about by slow feeding in a lethargic baby. Inappropriately high levels of insulin are the most likely cause of both the excess of fetal growth and the neonatal hypoglycaemia.

The infant of the insulin-dependent mother has an increased risk of having a major congenital abnormality. Apart from a rare developmental abnormality of the sacrum, no particular abnormalities are associated with maternal diabetes with a wide range of cardiac, neurological and skeletal defects reported.

The infant of the diabetic mother is also subject to additional problems, some of which are associated with maternal metabolic control but are also in part due to prematurity. Respiratory distress syndrome is one of the more serious but neonatal jaundice, polycythaemia and hypocalcaemia may also be found.

The overall outcome in pregnancy associated with maternal

diabetes is not as good as the general population for the infant of the insulin-dependent mother. Perinatal mortality in the major centres lies between 40 and 70 per thousand births. Approximately half the excess mortality is due to congenital malformations so that future improvements in the management of diabetic pregnancy depend upon a better understanding of this particular problem. The outcome in gestational diabetes, that is diabetes first diagnosed during pregnancy, is much better than in insulin-dependent diabetes because no excess of congenital malformations is found; the main problem in gestational diabetes being the large-for-dates infant.

Management

The aim of therapy should be to restore to as near normal physiological levels as possible, all the abnormal metabolism throughout the whole of pregnancy. Close cooperation between the physician's team, the obstetric and neonatal staff, and the patient is essential for the best results. Close attention to details is best achieved in joint clinics. Under these circumstances of intensive care, it is not always possible to be certain that one particular item of management is essential for a successful outcome. The outcome of diabetic pregnancy will be affected by the attitude of the patient because failure to attend for antenatal care and poor compliance with medical management will increase the risks. Some of the fault may be failure in patient education, sometimes the patient is incapable of understanding details of diabetic management, and sometimes the pregnancy is unwanted. In assessing risks for the individual patient the following should be considered:
a. the type of diabetes (established or gestational)
b. the clinical presence or absence of microvascular complications
c. cooperative or neglecting patient

Detection

Gestational diabetes is most often encountered in the third trimester when the greatest diabetogenic stress is present. Occasionally symptoms of diabetes will be found, but more

Table 6.1 Reasons for suspecting gestational diabetes

Previous large-for-dates baby (e.g. greater than 4.5 kg or 9.9 lb at term)
Significant glycosuria on at least two occasions
Family history-obesity and diabetes
Previous unexplained stillbirth

Table 6.2 Upper limits of normal during an oral glucose tolerance test in pregnancy

	Capillary blood glucose
Fasting	5.0 mmol/l
½ hour	10.0
1 hour	10.0
1½ hours	9.0
2 hours	8.0

often the diagnosis is made without symptoms as a result of careful screening in the antenatal population. The clinical clues towards diabetes are noted in Table 6.1.

A random blood glucose or blood glucose after a glucose load can be useful in screening for diabetes without waiting for a full glucose tolerance test, but it is difficult to standardise such procedures under busy routine antenatal care for the detection of impaired glucose tolerance in the whole antenatal population. The oral glucose tolerance test remains the definitive investigation for diabetes in pregnancy though the normal limits are not universally agreed. Using a 75 g oral load of glucose the upper limits of normal capillary blood glucose are suggested in Table 6.2.

Treatment

The aim of therapy is to maintain blood glucose levels as near normal as possible without causing clinical hypoglycaemia. Normal capillary fasting blood glucose levels are below 5 mmol/l and after meals below 7.5 mmol/l.

1. Diet

A review of the diet should be undertaken to ensure adequate calories and carbohydrate and a pint of milk a day. The 3 main meals should be reasonably balanced and snacks between meals, and particularly at bedtime, will be required by insulin-treated patients. The adequacy of diet can be monitored by observing a normal increase in body weight and the absence of fasting urine ketones. A full diet may be difficult early in pregnancy if severe anorexia or vomiting occur, and sometimes may be difficult in the last week or two of gestation.

2. Insulin

For the insulin-dependent patient, at least twice daily insulin will be needed during the second and third trimester. This should be given as a mixture of insulin of short and intermediate duration before breakfast and before the evening meal. Occasionally a longer-acting insulin in the evening or a third injection of intermediate insulin at bedtime is needed to ensure good metabolic control before breakfast. There is little change in insulin requirements in the first half of pregnancy, but from about the middle of the second trimester gradually increasing amounts of insulin are needed with approximately doubling of the dose by 36 weeks gestation. Increased insulin requirements are often noted during the administration of uterine muscle relaxing drugs such as ritodrine, isoxsuprine, orciprenaline and terbutaline, which are used in the inhibition of premature labour.

For the patient on oral hypoglycaemic drugs it is wise to use insulin during pregnancy to ensure optimum metabolic control. These drugs cross the placenta and in late pregnancy can result in fetal islet hypertrophy and neonatal hypoglycaemia. There is no evidence that the oral hypoglycaemic drugs are harmful in early pregnancy. For the patient controlled on diet alone, insulin should be used if blood glucose levels are consistently above the upper limit of normal.

On the day of a planned delivery, insulin can be given by continuous intravenous infusion of a short-acting insulin (2 units/hour), or by a small (12–16 units) sub-cutaneous dose of an intermediate duration insulin together with a 5 per cent dextrose intravenous infusion (1 litre in 8 hours). Therapy should be adjusted according to blood glucose monitoring. An intravenous infusion of 5 per cent dextrose is all that is usually required to manage diabetes following the spontaneous onset of labour. Immediately after delivery, insulin requirements fall and the patient can be maintained on her pre-pregnancy regimen if suitable.

Monitoring

Careful monitoring of diabetic control is an essential part of management of pregnancy complicated with maternal diabetes. The limited value of urine testing in general, and especially if the renal threshold is greatly lowered, should not deter its use in pregnancy. Most patients can achieve excellent metabolic control by testing four times a day. Home blood glucose monitoring is also of value, especially at bedtime and on rising, to help in adjusting therapy to avoid nocturnal hypoglycaemia, and to ensure adequate control of fasting blood glucose. Ideally antenatal attendance should be at a joint obstetric diabetic clinic every two weeks for a blood glucose check and careful assessment of fetal growth and development. Admission to hospital before delivery will depend on the degree of metabolic control achieved and whether any obstetric complications occur.

Contraception

The cooperation and effort required to maintain good metabolic control of diabetes comes best when pregnancy is planned. Contraceptive advice should be readily available to all diabetic women of child bearing age. Contraception for the diabetic patient should not differ greatly from that for the non-diabetic with the following guidelines:
a. contraception should be as effective as possible
b. oral contraception should not be used in the long-term once family size has been achieved because of the fear of aggravating arterial disease.
c. oral contraceptives may precipitate impaired glucose tolerance in a patient who has had gestational diabetes. Blood glucose will require checking in such patients.
d. once family size has been achieved it is reasonable to consider sterilisation. Normally two successful pregnancies provide enough problems for the diabetic to cope with as well as her own disease.

e. the presence of proliferative retinopathy and impaired renal function are not absolute contraindications to pregnancy but occasionally retinopathy deteriorates and in the long term the mother is less able to look after her family

f. the possibility of inheritance of diabetes is not generally considered a reason for avoiding pregnancy providing the father is non-diabetic. There is approximately 1 per cent risk of the infant of an insulin-dependent mother developing similar diabetes by the age of 25 years.

DIABETES IN CHILDREN

One of the first problems to deal with when a child is diagnosed with diabetes is the guilt feeling of the parents. Most diabetics at some time in their lives ask the question 'why me?' and this may be exceedingly acute in parents of young children who ask 'why our child?'. Most of the general public know that there is something to inheritance of diabetes and parents rapidly check their family tree for the disorder. Perhaps unconsciously they search for a source of 'faulty' genetic material but accept that they directly are responsible for passing it on. Careful explanation and reassurance are needed. To tell a parent immediately following diagnosis that they should assault their offspring with a needle and suffer cries and remorse in doing so, may not be the best manifestation of enthusiasm. In recent years, there has been considerable debate about where children should be treated initially. Proponents of home care argue that to take a child into hospital at this critical time may not be in the child's and parents' best interests and that teaching and stabilisation should be done at home. This argument has considerable emotive appeal but it is also clear in talking to parents that some are grateful for a period of hospital treatment of the child, giving the parents time to adjust and accept the diagnosis. As with much of diabetes there is no wrong way and no right way. Each family must be assessed and a decision made. The golden rule for the health care team must be to play to your strength. If resources in your area are concentrated into a strong, well-informed, community service then home care is a distinct possibility. If resources are hospital based then hospital care will follow logically. The safety of the patient is paramount and should never be only half met because of ideal-ogical persuasion that home care is best.

Once established, the management of diabetes is still not easy in this age group. Concepts of diabetic control will need modifying in 2 year olds. The management is then a gradual lesson in introducing independence. Injections should be the child's responsibility from as soon as they are able to learn; similarly urine or blood testing. Diet usually falls within the province of the mother. Special treats, so naturally given to other children such as ice cream, chocolate, and fizzy pops, may have to be withheld, but substitutes are always available in the way of fruit. Many of us are unconvinced that treats cannot be allowed, but would accept that a diet of crisps, pop, and sweets could be unacceptable. Simplicity is the keynote— plastic disposable syringes, urinary reagent sticks rather than clinitest, and clear straightforward advice which must always be non-conflicting. Beware the nurse saying one thing and the doctor another.

When old enough, nights away from home, school holidays abroad, or diabetic association camps should all be encour-aged in attempting to improve independence.

The child has special fears. Talking to children, ice cream deprivation may be accepted with equanimity but 'hypos' are not. Terrible fears exist that a hypo may occur during sleep and the child fail to wake up. Extra food may be taken before bed to avoid this. All too often this is followed by a trip to the doctor who increases the insulin in an attempt to improve overnight control. More food is eaten and a vicious circle is started. One of the most important features of the child's visit to the clinic is the height/weight check. Poor diabetic control during periods of rapid growth may stunt growth. Once the growth spurt is over, eating the same amount may lead to an increase in weight. A few years ago, the 'diabetic dwarf' was not uncommon, but with less strict dietary restriction and more attention to control, this syndrome is now extinct. To a large extent it has been replaced by the problem of the young, overweight, female who finds herself thus, just as she notices that there is another sex. Dieting is extraordinarily difficult for this group. Insulin and intake may need reduction in tandem and a few are successful in dieting. Better to prevent the problem before it arises. Exercise is important and forms part of the child's life from an early age, be it recreation or organised at school. Diabetics can do most exercise which their peers perform, but careful explanation to child, parents, and sometimes the school is often a good investment. It is generally accepted that planned exercise may be preceded by a reduction in insulin intake or an increase in carbohydrate. Neither precludes the necessity of carrying carbohydrate at all times. Simple advice, such as for mother to stitch a pocket into the patient's running shorts, should be stressed.

Paediatricians are often criticised for their care of the diabetic child. It is argued that poor diabetic control during childhood lays the foundation for disabling diabetic complications in later life. Since the paediatrician rarely sees such complications this may influence his care. This criticism is unjust and reflects a lack of understanding of the child's psychology by doctors and nurses treating adults. The paediatrician knows only too well how much a child will accept and how much the child with diabetes is being asked to accept. With a well-adjusted adult it may be acceptable for the health care team to concentrate on the disease. The paediatrician will invariably weigh this against the proper development of the child to an adult and have a more complete picture of what this involves. Nevertheless, diabetes does not constitute a subspecialty of paediatrics in the way it does of adult medicine since there are fewer patients. This should not imply that diabetic children should be spread around the district's paediatricians. Best results are obtained when knowledge and enthusiasm emit from the doctor. Personal pride prevents one paediatrician from accepting responsibility and the well-informed nurse may be the saving grace reaping rich rewards in preventing morbidity as adulthood supervenes.

DIABETES IN ADOLESCENTS

Adolescence is a time of rapid physical and psychological development and both may affect diabetic control and pose special problems. During adolescence, physical and sexual maturing takes place. Physical maturation is accompanied by the growth spurt with changes in hormonal secretory patterns and resultant metabolic effects.

The psychological changes which occur during adolescence are legion and it is perhaps surprising that most adolescents cope with the change. One of the fundamental developments which occur is in the relationship with parents. As a child the diabetic had no choice about attending a diabetic clinic and was usually accompanied by one or other parent. The adolescent may resent this continuing, as new found independence is sought. Parents may attempt to continue attending the clinic with the adolescent and often this is associated with the parents interest and role in looking after the diabetes. This is the time, however, when the diabetic has to learn to deal with his or her own disease and they should be encouraged to come to the clinic alone or at least should go through the consultation alone. Adult diabetic clinics with long waiting times and a population which includes blind diabetic patients and patients with amputations are far from ideal.

First attendance at an adolescent diabetic clinic is crucial since it sets the tone for the further relationship which will develop between staff and patient. Ideally, the adolescent needs staff with whom he or she can identify. In this respect, the medical staff should not be continually changing and the adolescent should be seen by someone they can come to know. There is little doubt that in our own clinic the most important member of the clinic staff is the nurse. The nurse, being the first member of staff to greet the patient, sets the whole tone of the clinic.

In adolescence social adjustment commences. The adolescent associates more and more with a group of similar people. Acceptance in a group brings considerable pressures to conform. Dress and other quickly changing fashions, which often bear the brunt of parental comment, are relatively unimportant compared with the lifestyle of the group. Eating habits may include fast foods and fizzy drinks, and later in adolescence there will be pressure to consume (often large quantities of) alcohol. The diabetic resents being the odd one out in the group who drinks low calorie drinks or diabetic lager. The need to take meals at specific times also marks him out. And overall, there is a constant threat of hypoglycaemia which may cause varying degrees of amazement, amusement, or ridicule in other group members.

Not surprisingly, some degree of resentment of diabetes is almost 'normal' in teenagers and this may manifest itself as absolute refusal to continue urine testing or giving only occasional sporadic injections. The task of the health care team in the community and in the clinic is to nurture the patient along, helping whenever and wherever possible and avoiding threatening reproaches or confrontations. It is better that the rebellious teenager visits the clinic regularly even if diabetic control horrifies the doctor, than they stop coming altogether, returning ten years later with advanced complications.

How strict should diabetic control be? Undoubtedly the answer is, as good as possible without alienating the patient by our attempts. Several studies have shown poor awareness of what is meant by control in adolescence. Absence of symptoms and paucity of hospital admissions may spell good control to the adolescent despite repeatedly raised blood glucoses or glycosylated haemoglobin concentration. That good control is more than this is a concept which needs gradual education and reinforcement. The means of obtaining good control may be the very thing we reach at the centre of the adolescent's rebellion. Injections are inconvenient, time-consuming and a constant reminder that the diabetic is different. Everything possible should be done to simplify the procedure. Clumsy glass syringes should be replaced by disposable plastic syringes. Swabbing of the skin with spirit has never been shown to be of any value except in making the skin more impenetrable.

BRITTLE DIABETES

Few aspects of insulin-dependent diabetes have aroused as much controversy as the concept of brittle diabetes. It is a rather loosely defined term taken to mean precipitous fluctuation between hyper- and hypoglycaemia. Many insulin-dependent diabetic patients pose this problem to a greater or lesser degree in their management. The term has been used by doctors to denote difficult-to-control diabetic patients. Patients seize on terms which mark them out from the rest of the clinic attenders, and when a patient says that Dr X told them they had brittle diabetes this may be more a reflection on the failure of the doctor, than the patient, to achieve adequate control. Brittle diabetes leads to an inability to lead a normal life because of diabetes, often with recurrent long periods of hospitalisation and if the term is to be used at all it should be used for these people.

A proportion of patients who undergo prolonged hospitalisation do so through manipulation of their disease. In this respect the diabetic has enormous power and may use it as an expression of dissatisfaction with home, school, or work. There is little doubt that increased environmental stress can provoke hyperglycaemia. Since stress is likely to fluctuate, an increase of insulin dosage at these times may result in hypoglycaemia a few days later.

No specific biochemical features of brittle diabetes have been found which would suggest that it is a distinct entity within insulin-dependent diabetes. No distinct psychological factors can be found in all patients, although systematic enquiries have not been made. They are likely to be unrewarding since it would be impossible to discern the basic personality from the effects of repeated hospitalisation.

Two factors deserve special attention. Brittle diabetics rarely die from the acute disturbance, although they may pay the price in later years. Most physicians would share with Dr John Malins the experience of talking with these patients in later years when the true extent of their manipulation may be heard.

What is the role of the nurse in all this? So-called brittle diabetics may latch on to one person, be it nurse or physician, and occupy extraordinary amounts of time. Diabetic control may improve—but it is nearly always temporary, until disillusionment sets in and a new nurse or physician is sought. No guidelines exist for how involved nurses should get, but when the nurse's life becomes disrupted that may be too high a price to pay.

Clearly there are 'brittle people' who have diabetes and will use the various aspects of the disorder for their own ends, to attract attention, avoid schooling or work and manipulate people. Over and above this are a very few patients who represent one end of the spectrum, from well-controlled to poorly-controlled patients. This may not be a distinct entity but they are the patients who develop ketoacidosis quickly, or may develop hypoglycaemia with small increases in insulin dosage. Perhaps this is what marks out such people from the remainder of our patients, that small changes in insulin dosage have a marked effect. Whether the patient benefits from the label 'brittle' is debatable, and if it induces a despairing reaction in the nurse and doctor it is counter-productive. When it marks the patient as someone with difficult diabetes, however, then early action if ketonuria develops, for example, may save the patient from unnecessary risk.

DIABETIC KETOACIDOSIS

Diabetic ketoacidosis is a severe life-threatening emergency with a mortality of 6–50 per cent. Mortalities as low as 6 per cent can be obtained only in centres which take a special interest in the condition and adopt an integrated team approach. Many versions of guidelines for treatment have been published but it should be clearly stated that none substitutes for careful nursing and medical care.

We are fortunate in having a specialised diabetic ward to which all ketoacidosis patients are admitted, but few centres see sufficient numbers of patients for this to be feasible. The advantages are that nursing staff and medical staff gain considerable experience in treating these patients. The concept of distributing patients in ketoacidosis throughout the general medical wards of a hospital, while giving many more medical and nursing staff a little experience, is probably not in the best interests of the patients. The seriousness of this condition merits care in an intensive therapy unit.

Less than 10 per cent of patients are in a coma at presentation and the term diabetic coma to describe this condition is not entirely appropriate. The majority will have some disturbance of consciousness ranging from sleepiness to aggressive confusion, but 20 per cent are fully alert and orientated. Diabetic ketoacidosis occurs as a result of insulin deficiency, with hyperglycaemia resulting from increased glucose production and decreased utilisation by tissues while fatty acids are released from fat cells and converted into ketone bodies by the liver. Hyperglycaemia results in polyuria and thirst, but satisfaction of the latter is unable to compensate for urinary losses and dehydration follows. Most patients will have lost more than 5 litres of body water and are also depleted of sodium, chloride, and potassium due to the osmotic diuresis. Vomiting may add to the water and electrolyte losses. The ketone bodies produced are acids and initially are buffered by bicarbonate. When the production exceeds the capacity to buffer the hydrogen ion, the pH of the blood falls. The commonest signs are the sweet smell of acetone on the breath and the acidotic respiration—rapid deep respirations called Kussmaul respiration. Some cases of ketoacidosis occur, therefore, in newly diagnosed insulin-deficient diabetics, and the remainder in established diabetic patients who err in their insulin regime either omitting insulin or reducing the dose, or through errors in administration.

In established diabetic patients an associated illness may lead to ketoacidosis. The commonest are infections, myocardial infarctions, or trauma. It is sad to hear of insulin-dependent diabetic patients who are advised to reduce their insulin dose when illness depresses appetite. Infections, for example, are associated with increased circulating concentrations of glucagon, cortisol, catecholamines, and growth hormone, and all these hormones have actions on metabolism antagonistic to insulin. Insulin requirement is thus increased. Measurements of blood or urinary glucose, and particularly ketonuria, are more important in this situation than an estimation of carbohydrate intake.

The aims of treatment are restoration of a normal clinical state and normal metabolism, and nurses play a major part in both.

Rehydration is extremely important and is usually undertaken with 0.9 per cent saline (154 mmol/1—previously called N for normal saline). Except in the elderly, rehydration is done rapidly initially. Urine flow should be checked to ensure that the patient does not have urinary retention. Dehydration is sometimes of a severity to lead to hypovolaemic shock and anuria. If either retention or anuria is present the patient should be catheterised. An important point in monitoring rehydration is to ensure that urinary losses do not exceed fluid infusion. Infusion of saline may increase serum sodium to an unacceptably high level when 'half normal' saline (77 mmol/1) may be needed. The main danger of rapid rehydration in other than young patients is cardiac failure. A central venous pressure line is useful in these circumstances and frequent measurement should be charted.

Along with rehydration potassium is replaced. Although there is a total body deficit of potassium, serum potassium may be markedly elevated. This is measured frequently during treatment but a good guide is in the ECG. The height of the T wave, particularly in lead II, should be examined. If it is higher than the complex, hyperkalaemia is present. Flat T waves denote hypokalaemia. The ECG is monitored during treatment and it is more readily and quickly available than serum potassium measurement. Depending on the serum potassium or the ECG, 10–40 mmol of potassium are added to each infusion bottle. It is important that after adding the potassium to the infusion fluid, the contents are mixed thoroughly, otherwise the patient may receive a potentially lethal concentration of potassium with the first few mls of infusion fluid.

Rapid-acting insulin is always used to treat ketoacidosis. So called low-dose regimens are the treatment of choice, and older high dose regimens imply a reactionary physician. Erudite arguments persist amongst physicians regarding intramuscular or intravenous regimens, but the soundest advice is to use the regimen which is safest for the level of nursing and medical care. Experience suggests that less can go wrong with intramuscular regimens. The intramuscular insulin injection usually falls to the nurse to administer and in this regard it should be realised that timing is exceedingly important. Hourly intramuscular injections means hourly. Blood glucose is monitored hourly with reagent stix. A few patients may not respond to the treatment initially, and since reagent stix have disadvantages at high glucose levels, laboratory measurement should be undertaken in the early stages.

When blood glucose falls to 14 mmol/1 infusion of glucose (5 per cent dextrose) is commenced and either intramuscular insulin is less frequent or subcutaneous insulin (4 hourly) is commenced.

A feature of diabetic ketoacidosis is abdominal pain and a large distended stomach. This can contain litres of fluid and in comatose or semi-conscious patients gastric aspiration should be performed. Since in semi-conscious patients a gag reflex, although diminished, may be present, aspiration during passing of a tube should be avoided. If the PO_2 while breathing air is less than 11 KPa (80 mmHg) oxygen should be given.

Routine nursing care should be given. The word routine is an anathema since there are good reasons for certain acts. Occasionally during ketoacidosis and its treatment, peripheral nerves may be damaged leading particularly to foot-drop. This occurs in the most severe cases and is avoidable. Similarly, particularly in the elderly, peripheral ischaemic events occur. During treatment, areas, other than the head and neck which protrude above the bed clothes, should be regularly inspected. Some centres favour low dose heparinisation for high risk patients. Infusion of blood or plasma is rarely needed in severely shocked patients. Treatment of the precipitating cause of ketoacidosis is most important. Infections account for 30–50 per cent of episodes of diabetic ketoacidosis and should receive enthusiastic antibiotic therapy. At presentation, pyrexia is often not a feature and indeed severe hypothermia may be present. This should be treated with gradual warming of the patient, but the large volumes of infusion fluids may have a distinct cooling effect which can readily be counteracted by warmers.

Bicarbonate infusion is a controversial point with advantages and disadvantages. Since severe acidosis may have deleterious effects on cardiovascular, respiratory and nervous systems, it is suggested that bicarbonate be given if the pH is less than 7.1. Not more than 150 mmol should be given without assessment of the effect upon pH. It should be given in the weakest solution stocked by the hospital (preferably 1.2 per cent). Bicarbonate results in a fall in serum potassium as does insulin administration, and hypokalaemia must be avoided or arrhythmias are likely and sometimes fatal. This is further reason for ECG monitoring.

The mortality of ketoacidosis may be divided into two parts. Firstly, it is associated with a precipitating illness, e.g. septicaemia or myocardial infarction. Good nursing care can reduce this mortality to a small degree, although prevention in the community or early detection is all important. A proportion of the mortality, however, arises during treatment and may be termed preventable. The death of a 20-year-old in ketoacidosis from hypokalaemia or another preventable cause, rightly casts gloom and despondency at the tragic loss.

HYPEROSMOLAR NON-KETOTIC DIABETIC COMA

Considerably less common than diabetic ketoacidosis but carrying a higher mortality of around 50 per cent is the condition of hyperosmolar non-ketotic diabetic coma. The name is good one denoting the essential features of the condition. The blood glucose concentration may be exceedingly high (greater than 60 mmol/1) while blood urea, sodium, potassium, and other ions are all elevated. Despite these biochemical abnormalities, ketone bodies are not a predominant feature of the condition, although small amounts may be present in the blood or urine which are insufficient to result in ketoacidosis.

The reasons underlying the development of the condition are unknown. In our own clinical practice, two groups of patients predominantly develop hyperosmolar coma. They are the elderly and some West Indian patients. The usual history is of the development of thirst which the patient attempts to relieve by drinks high in sugar such as lucozade or Coca-cola. These enhance the hyperglycaemia, and polyuria and dehydration are major features. As large amounts of body water are lost, the effects of dehydration are seen both in the biochemical abnormalities and in the disturbance of consciousness which may progress to coma.

It is suggested that these patients are not totally insulin-deficient but retain sufficient circulating insulin to inhibit ketone body formation from non-esterified fatty acids. This is supported by the later finding that after successful treatment of the acute episode, many of these patients may be treated successfully with oral hypoglycaemic agents or dietary therapy. This is in stark contrast to patients presenting with ketoacidosis, which implies severe insulin deficiency and in therapeutic terms, a lifetime of insulin injections.

With low-dose insulin regimens, the treatment of hyperosmolar coma is similar to that of ketoacidosis initially, i.e. hourly short-acting insulin. The major difference lies in the choice of rehydrating fluid. Clearly, if the patient's serum sodium is greater that 160 mmol/1 it follows logically that rehydration with $\frac{1}{2}$N saline which contains 77 mmol/1 of sodium is preferred to rehydration with 154 mmol/1 saline. The infusion of hypotonic solutions, however, is not without certain dangers, particularly that of haemolysis. It is probably wise to set a limit of a maximum of 2 litres of hypotonic saline. The remainder of the management is as for diabetic ketoacidosis with emphasis upon the special care of elderly patients. A central venous pressure line is a useful guide to rehydration while the viscous nature of the blood results in the risk of thrombotic episodes.

INFECTION AND SURGERY

Infection

Infection may result in secretion of hormones into the blood which oppose the action of insulin upon tissues. Glucagon, growth hormone, corticosteroids, and catecholamines may all be implicated. To obtain the same degree of metabolic control, therefore, more insulin is required during infection. The important point is that this is true even when the infection is associated with loss of appetite.

Occasionally, however, an infection may not result in loss of control. The practical rule is that blood or urine tests should be monitored rather more than appetite. Persistently raised blood glucose or glycosuria indicate that more insulin is needed. Since the hormonal response to infection not only acts to raise blood glucose but also to produce more ketones, the urine should be monitored for ketonuria. Heavy ketonuria implies imminent ketoacidosis even if glycosuria is not heavy. Vomiting in patients taking insulin is difficult to manage at home and, indeed, may be the first sign of ketoacidosis. Advice is best sought early, especially when ketoacidosis is a risk. Dehydration from polyuria is a sign that you have delayed too long. Dry tongue, sunken eye balls, and loss of the elastic nature of the skin are all useful signs of dehydration.

Insulin-dependent diabetic patients should be taught correctly how to deal with an infection. In part, this involves explanation of changes in insulin dose but also when to seek help. Heavy ketonuria or vomiting are mandatory signs that help is needed. It is sometimes useful to omit long-acting insulins during a bad infection and give short-acting insulin four to six times a day. Blood or urine may be tested before each injection and the dose adjusted. A dose should not be omitted because the results look good. Frequent, small amounts are needed until the depot insulin is reintroduced.

Beware of urine reagent tests which give falsely low estimates of glycosuria when ketonuria is present.

Surgery

Good control of diabetes during and after surgery may help to promote wound healing. The significance of this is often played down by anaesthetists or surgeons who particularly want to avoid hypoglycaemia.

Patients on diet or oral agents, undergoing minor surgery, may be managed simply by omitting the oral agent on the day of operation, although some tablets with long half-lives may need to be omitted on the day before operation. The patient may need to be warned in advance of this. For occasional patients on insulin, undergoing minor surgery, the morning insulin may be delayed until the first post-surgery meal.

If in doubt, and during major surgery, insulin should be given. Numerous regimens exist for this whereby a fraction (half or a third) of the daily dose is given pre-surgery (as rapid or as intermediate-acting insulin), and some dextrose is given during surgery, either by bolus or infusion. There is little doubt that an infusion of insulin gives best results and is easily managed. This can be given by infusion pump (0.5 units–2 units/h) or can be added to an infusion of glucose. This latter technique has the advantage that if for any reason dextrose infusion ceases, insulin infusion also ceases. The infusion can be continued immediately post-operatively until eating recommences. The technique is therefore particularly suitable for gastrointestinal surgery.

Dextrose (500 ml of 5 per cent) has quick-acting insulin (5–10 units) added. Insulin binds to plastic or glass bottles and giving sets and this can be nullified by discarding the first 50 ml which saturates the binding sites. Thereafter, the infusion is run at

100 ml/h and blood glucose monitored. Lowering or increasing the amount of insulin added on the basis of blood glucose measurement may be necessary. It is no longer necessary, using this technique, for the diabetic patient to go first on an operating list—indeed a run-up to the operation of a couple of hours may allow the finding of the rate of infusion needed to obtain and maintain normal blood glucose levels.

A similar technique may be used for the management of labour or Caesarian section.

A special problem arises in what has been labelled 'the diabetic abdomen'. Abdominal pain is not uncommon in ketoacidosis and does not imply a surgically treatable lesion in the abdomen. It usually resolves soon after starting treatment and it does not occur without heavy ketonuria. An intra-abdominal infection, however, may also precipitate ketoacidosis and the latter will be difficult to treat until, for example, the infected appendix is removed. Under these circumstances rehydration and insulin are used immediately and surgery should follow rapidly with acceptance that diabetic control is not good but is a compromise between the need to treat the ketoacidosis and the need to treat the cause of ketoacidosis.

HYPOGLYCAEMIA (see also Ch. 4)

The symptoms and effects of low blood glucose are potentially serious. A proper understanding, early recognition and prompt treatment of hypoglycaemia are vital aspects in the education of diabetic patients. This education must include all patients on insulin treatment, immediate members of an insulin-dependent patient's family and all health professionals. Hypoglycaemia is often known by the patient as a hypoglycaemic or insulin reaction or attack, or simply as a 'hypo'. Hypoglycaemia is an inevitable risk of all types of insulin treatment. Hypoglycaemia is unusual but can occur on sulphonylurea drugs, particularly if the patient stops eating or develops renal failure.

The symptoms of hypoglycaemia are partly due to lack of glucose for the nervous system (neuroglycopenia) and partly due to sympathetic nervous and adrenaline response (adrenergic) (Table 6.3). The particular pattern of symptoms varies

Table 6.3 Clinical features of hypoglycaemia

Sympathetic nervous system	Central nervous system
Sweating	Tingling around mouth and in fingers
Pallor	Sinking feeling
Rapid pulse	Double vision
Anxiety	Tremor
	Strange or drunken behaviour
	Weakness and unsteadiness
	Light headedness
	Drowsiness
	Early morning headache
	Fits
	Coma

from person to person, but with an individual tends to be fairly constant from one episode to another. Some change in symptoms may be experienced in the patient with longstanding diabetes (see section on Autonomic neuropathy). The symptom of straightforward hunger is unusual, but a sinking feeling in the stomach is common. A change in behaviour is an early warning sign for those closely associated with the insulin-dependent patient. Such behaviour may be unusual flippancy, obstinacy or aggression. This, in turn, may obstruct the treatment of a hypoglycaemic episode. The usual symptoms of hypoglycaemia are rapid in onset over several minutes. The rare patient who has absolutely no early warning symptoms is at a great disadvatage in managing their diabetes with current insulin methods. One of the fears of patients is having an episode of hypoglycaemia at night and not waking up. Nocturnal hypoglycaemia is in fact not uncommon, but often wakes the patient or disturbs another member of the household. More careful monitoring of blood glucose has shown that self-limiting hypoglycaemia may occur while the patient is asleep without disturbing him. On waking, urinary incontinence may have occurred or a headache may be present.

The dangers of hypoglycaemia for the patient are the injuries that may occur while semi- or unconscious, such as falls or burns, and occasionally brain damage is so severe that the patient does not recover consciousness and hypoglycaemia is fatal. The danger of hypoglycaemia for others is largely related to accidents at work or while driving where third parties can be involved.

Diagnosis

Hypoglycaemia must be the first consideration on seeing any unconscious diabetic patient. The patient usually appears pale and sweaty. Most episodes need not be confirmed by taking a blood glucose test, but this may be useful in doubtful cases with a history of funny turns, or when the history is not known in semi-conscious or comatose patients. The blood glucose level in symptomatic hypoglycaemia is usually less than 2 mmol/l. It is often confusing for the patients who rely on urine testing to find glycosuria at the same time as hypoglycaemia. Little reliance should be placed on the finding of glycosuria at this time as the bladder may contain urine excreted several hours previously when the blood glucose level may have been much higher. It is also quite common to find significant glycosuria sometime after hypoglycaemia which may in part be due to overtreatment, or in some instances due to the secretion of counter-regulatory hormones (Somogyi effect).

Treatment

The risk of hypoglycaemia can be reduced considerably by paying due attention to certain general principles (Table 6.4).Wherever possible, treatment of hypoglycaemia (Table 6.5) should be by carbohydrate taken by mouth. Mild hypoglycaemic symptoms should respond to 10 g of carbohydrate, but if symptoms are not relieved within ten minutes a further 10–20 g should be taken. If the patient is unable to swallow, an intramuscular injection of glucagon is often successful in relieving hypoglycaemia partially. Glucagon may take 20

Table 6.4 Management of hypoglycaemia

Prevention
Take regular and adequate meals
Monitor metabolic control
Adjust diet and/or insulin according to physical activity
Avoid excess alcohol
Avoid sudden changes of species of insulin
Carry carbohydrate

Table 6.5 Management of hypoglycaemia

Treatment	
Oral	
10 g carbohydrate	3 glucose tablets
	1 tablespoon Ribena
	2 tablespoon Lucozade
	2 teaspoon sugar in water, milk or juice
Intramuscular injection	
1 mg glucagon	
Intravenous injection	
50% dextrose	

minutes to have an effect and as soon as the patient can swallow further carbohydrate should be taken by mouth to prevent relapse. If the patient is unable to swallow and glucagon is unavailable, an intravenous injection of 50 per cent glucose solution is required. While help is being summoned, simple care of the unconscious patient can avoid serious inhalation problems or self-inflicted injuries.

DIABETES IN THE ELDERLY

As has been seen in discussing aetiology and types of diabetes, the majority of newly diagnosed elderly diabetic patients can be treated with a diet or suitable oral agents. However, there are a number of special problems which face this age-group.

Diagnosis may be a problem. The majority of diabetics admitted with hyperosmolar coma are elderly, and result from delay in diagnosis, either by the patient failing to seek advice or undue delay having sought advice. Once diagnosed, the problem to be faced is identical to that of adolescence. How strict should diabetic control be? There is no clear-cut answer to this question. Most physicians are prepared to relax standards of control in this age-group, accepting poor control on oral agents or on insulin provided the patient is symptom-free. The social inconvenience and dependency are often considered negative factors to starting an elderly patient on insulin. It is certainly true that new skills such as injection technique are usually difficult to learn at this age. Symptoms, however, may be difficult to assess and a lack of complaint of classical symptoms does not preclude an increased sense of well-being on changing from being poorly controlled on oral agents to insulin. One thing the nurse should never do, is assume that all elderly patients will not learn injection technique, and an attempt should always be made when the possibility exists.

The diabetic patient taking insulin and growing old gracefully may also be experiencing failure in eyesight and dexterity. To become dependent upon someone for injections is a sad blow to these people and the full range of gadgets simplifying the procedure warrant a trial (Ch. 5).

The elderly by virtue of age are a high risk group for peripheral vascular disease and other complications. The snip of a toe nail which goes wrong may be all that is needed to start the rot which ends in above or below knee amputation and immobility. Failing eyesight may be the cause and this should be remembered. It is much easier to ask the patient about their feet than to actually inspect them. It is also rather pointless if early damage was not obvious to the patient because of poor eyesight, or if it was in an area not regularly viewed by the patient, e.g. the sole of the foot.

Once tissue damage is present this may be taken as an indication to improve diabetic control. There is a school of opinion that argues, that since the elderly are an at-risk group for complications, and since control affects the development of complications, it is inadequate to accept a relaxation of standards of control. The theory of this argument cannot be faulted but many times in practice it is untenable. The risk of hypoglycaemia in the elderly person living alone, who may be careless on diet or mildly confused, is enormous.

Who should look after elderly diabetics, the family practitioner or the hospital clinic? A caring family practitioner with practice-based nurses can do the job best. Many patients actually seem to enjoy their visits to the hospital, however, and in these the clinic has a role in promoting well-being. The diabetic who has attended regularly for 20 years cannot suddenly be told that they need no longer come. Sharing care between the hospital and community is a logical step, but this should not simply be a duplication of care and conflicting advice. Because of this, the community nurse has a major role. Regular inspection of the feet, reminders of diet, and detection of problems early, fall within their orbit. All may reap rich rewards for the patient in minimising morbidity and preserving independence.

DIABETES AMONGST IMMIGRANTS

Just as diabetes is a syndrome and cannot be considered a single disease, so an immigrant cannot be considered as a single problem. Patients from different genetic backgrounds will bring different types of diabetes. The main difference being the relative rarity of insulin-dependent diabetes in some groups and the frequency of obesity-associated diabetes in other groups. Patients from different cultural backgrounds will bring different problems to the adjustments required for managing diabetes. These may be educational, especially if there is a major language difference, when the spoken word through an interpreter may be the only means of teaching about diabetes. Dietary differences are less of a problem now that high unrefined carbohydrate diets have been shown to be satisfactory for optimum metabolic control. The main difficulty in our society, regardless of ethnic background, is the difficulty in controlling obesity. The indications and acceptance of insulin treatment are not different in the immigrant, and it is expected that the use of human insulin will overcome the rare objection to porcine or bovine insulin, made for religious reasons. Fasting for religious reasons is no problem in the diet-alone treated patient, but problems of hypoglycaemia may arise in the tablet or insulin treated patient unless adjustments are made to therapy. Such patients should be advised to seek permission not to fast for prolonged periods.

EMPLOYMENT OF DIABETIC PATIENTS

Employment is a major concern for the insulin-dependent diabetic patient. Strict rules regarding employment would be unfair when there is such a wide variation from patient to patient with how they cope with their disorder. Similarly many patients on once or twice daily injections have successful careers in surprisingly difficult jobs.

The major concern of the patient, the employer, and the

doctor is hypoglycaemia. If unrecognised, this may result in a change in behaviour or drowsiness. Even if recognised, the worry is that unconsciousness may supervene before adequate treatment begins. It will be a source of concern if such an episode endangers the patient working with heavy machinery, or other workers, or the general public.

In view of this, certain employments are considered unsuitable for patients receiving insulin treatment. They are not allowed to hold a Heavy Goods Vehicle Licence or to drive Public Service Vehicles. Insulin-dependent diabetes is normally a bar to the fire services or the armed or police forces. We should stress, however, that these authorities are often both considerate and compassionate to the person who enters one of the forces and then at a later date develops insulin-dependent diabetes. The diagnosis does not necessarily imply an end to the patient's career in, for example, a police force.

A number of employments are potentially dangerous for an insulin-dependent patient. Such jobs as working as a steeplejack or window cleaner or on scaffolding would not normally be considered ideal. Rather more debatable are jobs involving the supervision of heavy machinery. We should add that some employers' own insurance schemes may exclude these patients because of the premium loading imposed to cover the higher risk of mortality in insulin-dependent diabetic patients. We would probably think that in an ideal world, regular hours of work would be most suitable for patients taking insulin. With this in mind we might conclude that jobs involving considerable road travel with overnight stays away from home and meals in hotels or restaurants, would not be entirely suitable for our patients. Clearly it would be unacceptable to state this as a general rule since a number of diabetic patients do indeeded cope with such problems without detriment to their diabetes. In similar manner, many diabetic patients work shifts and will require advice on manipulation of their insulin injections when starting or ending a period of shift work. This is not usually a problem in patients taking two injections daily where simple advice on manipulation of dose should be given. In this situation two injections per day is preferrable to a single daily injection. A patient working the final night of a period of night shifts may take their insulin before going to work, work a full night, and then revert to a daytime existence. It is sensible to reduce the dose of insulin given for the final night and recommence the normal daily dose next morning. Similar manipulation will be necessary at the start of night shifts.

We must encourage our insulin-dependent diabetic patients to be honest in declaring their disorder to potential employers. In addition, it is important for the diabetic patient to tell his colleagues at work, in order that they can assist in the early recognition and management of hypoglycaemia. This will also help to aid understanding of the diabetic patient's need for regular meal breaks and snacks.

Diabetes is a registerable disability and registration may be helpful for problems of re-employment. The British Diabetic Association have a wide experience of problems encountered by diabetics seeking employment. They are always prepared to give well-founded advice and if they think an employer's decision unjust, to take up the case on the patient's behalf with that employer.

NEW APPROACHES TO TREATMENT

From time to time reports appear in the popular press of new treatment for diabetes. Such reports are often latched on to by certain groups of patients. These include patients with a good grasp of the significance of diabetes and particularly the problems it may pose for them in later life. They are usually aware of the prevailing attitude that good control of diabetes prevents or retards the development of complications. Thus any report which indicates a new means of improving diabetic control is avidly read in preparation for the questions at the next visit to the diabetic clinic. A second group of patients who take notice of new developments are those who would do almost anything to avoid the daily ritual of injections.

It is usually the case that reports of new treatments appear prematurely, and the distinction is not often drawn between techniques of treatment with research applications, and treatments which will eventually find their way into the therapeutic armamentarium. Often the development of a research tool into a new form of treatment takes many years, and careful explanation to the patient that the technique may not be widely applicable for some years must be done with tact and care in order to avoid disappointment and disillusionment.

Some of the techniques outlined below have strict limitations of applicability, while others will need many years of further research work before any widespread clinical use can be envisaged. Perhaps amongst the most promising of recent developments are the use of open-loop systems and the potential use of closed-loop systems.

Loop systems

The increase in insulin secretion in response to a rise in blood glucose concentration and the subsequent fall in secretion as blood glucose is lowered, is an example of a closed-loop system. As was described in Chapter 2, this loop is broken in the insulin-dependent diabetic patient. Thus current treatment of insulin-dependent diabetes involves the administration of subcutaneous depots of insulin. The release of insulin from the depot is determined mainly by the physical form of the administered insulin and it is without regard, therefore, to the prevailing concentration of glucose in the blood. To replace this closed-loop system in the insulin-dependent diabetic patient we would have to obtain a constant measurement of blood glucose and an infusion system which responds to changes in this blood glucose, infusing greater or lesser amounts of insulin. This would constitute an artificial closed-loop system and indeed many groups of research workers and some commercial interests have already developed such a system.

An open-loop system consists of an infusion device which can infuse variable amounts of insulin. In such a system the afferent limb of the loop, that is constant blood glucose monitoring, is not included. Many research groups have extensive experience of open-loop systems using subcutaneous insulin infusion.

We should just add that the distinction between an open and a closed loop system may be blurred. For example, a variable subcutaneous insulin infusion may be adjusted in response to repeated blood glucose monitoring using reagent sticks or meters. In this the true closed-loop system, continuous glucose measurement—a computer to calculate insulin infusion rates in response to these measurements—an infusion system controlled by the computer, is replaced by a considerably cruder closed-loop system, intermittent blood glucose measurement—the human brain which calculates infusion rates—and a variable rate infusion system.

Subcutaneous insulin infusions

Of the techniques described in this section most experience has been gained with subcutaneous insulin infusions. In England this work has been pioneered by Professor Harry Keen and his group at Guy's Hospital in London.

The object of the system is to make available in the diabetic patient, insulin concentrations which are appropriate for the level of the blood glucose. To do this a constant basal infusion is given to mimic the constant basal secretion of insulin in non-diabetic subjects, and at meal times the rate of infusion is increased to cover the meal eaten. Since there is no continuous measurement of blood glucose in this open-loop system the rate of insulin infusion must be determined empirically. With experience it is possible to anticipate, with a fair degree of accuracy, the insulin requirement needed both basally and to cover mealtimes. The majority of pumps available are capable of delivering two distinct rates of insulin infusion. Simpler pumps, which deliver at a single rate, and more sophisticated pumps, which can be extensively pre-programmed, are available. With pumps that deliver at two rates, adjustment of the basal insulin infusion can only be done by dilution of the insulin preparation. The reservoir of diluted insulin which the pump drives into the patient is, in the majority of cases, contained in a syringe.

Short-acting insulin is always used with a pump. The insulin is delivered via a small cannula or a butterfly needle which is inserted into a subcutaneous site. Usually the anterior abdominal wall is used, although the upper arm has also been used. The subcutaneous cannula, or needle, should be re-sited frequently, but this can often be done by the patient.

There is little doubt that good control of blood glucose concentration can be obtained using this system. There are drawbacks, however, particularly with regard to the infusion sites. Local infection and allergy may occur, although this is not common. Of rather more serious potential is the dislodging of the cannula. During the day this may be replaced by the patient. However, if it occurs during sleep the patient may receive no insulin for a number of hours and blood glucose may rise rapidly. In addition, certain mechanical aspects of the pump may fail. In view of this, a number of alarm systems have been incorporated in most of the pumps which will signal a motor fault, empty reservoir, or low battery. Unfortunately, it is far less easy to introduce an alarm system which would be triggered by dislodgement of the infusion cannula.

Patients who are suitable for continuous subcutaneous insulin infusion must be chosen carefully. The technique demands a high level of motivation from the patient. It does allow the patient a greater flexibility of life style, particularly with regard to meal times. In return, however, special precautions have to be taken when bathing, and the size and weight of currently available pumps sometimes evokes adverse comment.

As an alternative to subcutaneous infusion other routes of administration have been tried. Less experience has been gained with intramuscular, intravenous and intra-peritoneal infusions.

As an introduction to subcutaneous infusion we would recommend a small booklet entitled *Infusion Pumps and Insulin Therapy* published and obtainable from Novo Laboratories Limited.

Closed-loop systems

The closed-loop system of glucose sensor, computer, and infusion system has been called an 'artificial pancreas'. A more correct title is a glucose-controlled insulin infusion system. In the system, blood is continuously withdrawn from a peripheral vein of the patient. The blood passes to a glucose sensor which continuously measures blood glucose concentration. The results of this are fed to a computer and this can be programmed to maintain blood glucose in the patient at a desired level. In order to do this the computer controls an infusion pump, and insulin is infused through a second intravenous cannula. The computer is programmed to infuse greater amounts of insulin in response to a rise in blood glucose concentration and to decrease the insulin infusion in response to a fall.

There is no doubt that using this system blood glucose concentration in an insulin-dependent diabetic patient may be restored to normal for as long as the patient is attached to the machine. The great disadvantage to date is the size of the machine which approximates to the size of a colour television set. This means that patients may be attached to the artificial pancreas for only a limited time. It would be true to say that this system has not found a routine clinical use but does have some investigational possibilities. It is unlikely that further developments of a closed-loop system will occur until a greater degree of miniaturisation can be achieved.

We should add that it is possible to achieve considerable sophistication in the miniaturisation of infusion pumps. What is more difficult at the present time is to develop a reliable, small glucose sensor. The problems of continuously sampling blood for measurement of blood glucose concentration from a peripheral vein are numerous and it is likely that the development of a glucose sensor would have to depend upon a non-invasive method of measuring glucose.

Oral insulin

It is unusual for a nurse or doctor not to be asked at some time in their career about oral insulin. Insulin is a protein. Proteins which are introduced into the gastrointestinal tract are digested to their constituent amino acids. Thus, if insulin were to be given orally, digestion of the hormone would take place. One way round this is to protect the insulin through the digestion and absorption processes. A number of ways have been tried to achieve this end. The most promising is to surround the insulin by an envelope of fat. In this way the package may escape digestion and be absorbed. The insulin can then be released following breakdown of the fatty envelope.

It has been adequately shown that insulin can be absorbed and released in this manner. To date however it has proved impossible to obtain a consistency of absorption and release.

This means that the amount of insulin released from a given dose of oral insulin is exceedingly variable. This limits further development of oral insulin preparations.

Transplantation of the pancreas

Transplantation of the pancreas into an insulin-dependent diabetic patient cannot be undertaken in the same way as transplantation of other organs. Renal transplantation for example is undertaken when kidney failure is a direct threat to the life of the patient. We cannot make the same claims for the insulin-dependent diabetic patient and his pancreas. The insulin-dependent diabetic patient can live a relatively normal life provided regular injections of insulin are taken. Thus, unless the risks of pancreatic transplantation were extremely low, or a diabetic patient was having transplantation of another organ, it would be difficult to propose a case for pancreatic transplantation. The pancreas has proved to be a difficult organ to transplant. In part, this is due to its function as an organ of digestion. The pancreas produces enzymes which are important in digestion of food-stuffs in the gastrointestinal tract. Given the opportunity, these enzymes will not only digest food but will digest the patient's own tissues. In addition, as with other transplanted organs, rejection of the organ is an important consideration.

A small number of transplants of the pancreas have been performed in insulin-dependent diabetic patients, usually accompanying a kidney transplant for end-stage diabetic nephropathy. Results are only moderately good, and at present there would have to be exceptional circumstances present before a pancreas transplant would be considered.

Islet cell transplantation

As an alternative to transplanting a whole pancreas, experiments in animals have shown that transplantation of the islets of Langerhans is a real possibility. Since, in the insulin-dependent diabetic patient, what we are attempting to replace by transplantation is secretion of insulin, it would appear logical to transplant mainly those cells which are responsible for this. In animals, islets of Langerhans can be obtained from one animal and inserted into a diabetic animal via the portal vein or under the capsule of the spleen. The cells will remain alive and both produce insulin and secrete it, in response to an appropriate stimulus. The technique is so successful that the previously diabetic animal reverts to a normal animal.

We should not imagine, however, that the technique is totally devoid of problems. The islets for transplantation must be obtained from some source, and while this can be done by sacrificing one animal for another experimentally, obtaining human islets would be a major problem. In addition, the rejection which may occur with all transplanted organs may occur also with transplanted islets of Langerhans.

Conclusion

Research workers in diabetes are constantly searching for techniques which will allow us to improve diabetic control. It must be a source of comfort to the diabetic patient, and to all who care for the diabetic patient, that such enthusiastic and extensive work is taking place. The search for ways of improving diabetic control rests on the firm belief that this will prevent or retard the development of the long-term, disabling complications of diabetes. It is likely that the development and application of these techniques will demand much more of our abilities to educate the diabetic patient.

Further reading and information

Borger R, Seaborne A E M 1982 The psychology of learning. Penguin Books, Harmondsworth

Carbohydrate countdown, The British Diabetic Association, 10 Queen Anne Street, London W1M OBD

Insulin pumps and insulin therapy. Novo Laboratories Limited, Ringway House, Bell Road, Daneshill East, Basingstoke, Hants RG24 OGN

Mann J, Oxford Diabetic Group 1982 The diabetics diet book. Martin Dunitz, London

Nurse G 1980 Counselling and the Nurse, 2nd edn. Harvey Miller & Metcalf, London

Paul A A, Southgate D A T 1978 McCance and Widdowson's The composition of foods. HMSO/Elsevier

Rogers J 1977 Adults learning, 2nd edn. Open University Press, Milton Keynes

World Health Organization Expert Committee on Diabetes Mellitus 1980 World Health Organization, Geneva

Index